- Revi

"A poignant and well needed collective account of 12 women's experiences of surgical menopause. Patients experiencing induced menopause are more often than not overlooked by their surgeons who have little interest or awareness on the 'what' next. This book helps fill the gaps. With invaluable advice on preparing for surgery and self-care tips for both immediately after surgery and longer-term, as well as signposting to support, women can feel more empowered through menopause and start operating at their new optimum. Every woman considering or embarking on surgery that will induce menopause should read this!"
Lesley Salem
Founder, Over the Bloody Moon

"This book is fantastic"
Hayley Cockman
Premature-menopause advocate

"Real stories from real women sharing the truth that surgical menopause is indeed difficult and intense, but with time, we can move from feeling fragile and vulnerable to capable and confident"
Lori Ann King
Author of 'Come Back Strong: Balanced Wellness after Surgical Menopause'

"They say the best way to learn is by personal experience. But what if you're so ensconced in hormonal hideousness that you can't string a sentence together let alone research what the heck is happening to you. Surgical menopause is not a common topic even among regular menopause conversations. There's not much real-life literature about it either. This book is vital. These stories are of real women who've gone through surgical menopause. Tough for most, manageable for a few. You will hear intimate and detailed accounts that will reassure, support and help you through yours. Hold on, it might be a bumpy ride!"
Sam Bunch
Author of 'Menopause - A Hot Topic' and 'Collecting Conversations'

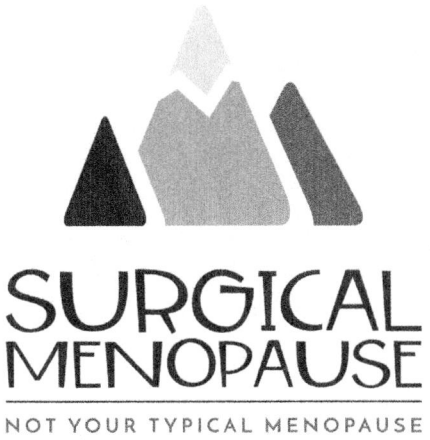

NOT YOUR TYPICAL MENOPAUSE

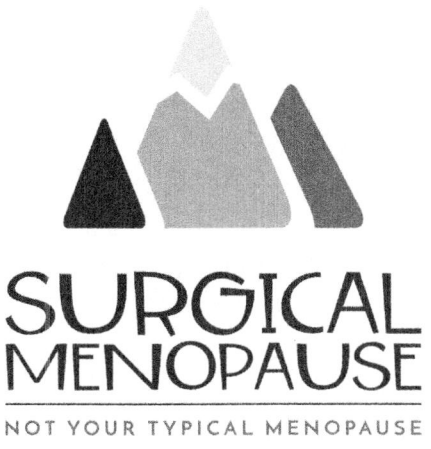

SURGICAL
MENOPAUSE

NOT YOUR TYPICAL MENOPAUSE

Edited by Helen Kemp

For surgical menopause warriors everywhere.
We see you, we salute you.

Contents

Introduction

I know what you're thinking. Here's yet another book about menopause, banging on about HRT, vaginal dryness and hot flushes. You may have a point about another book, to which I say "hooray". Knowledge is power and forewarned is indeed forearmed when it comes to our health. If one single woman is helped by this book, it will have been worth it.

I believe surgical menopause is different when compared to natural menopause. It can feel brutal. Even more so when it occurs at a young age. Yet women seldom receive accurate information prior to, or even after surgery. How is it we can have a significant chunk of our endocrine system removed, only to be sent on our way with advice not to lift anything heavier than a kettle for six weeks, and to abstain from sex for the same duration?

From my own lived experience and from hearing women's experiences up and down the country, I know how often surgical menopause completely floors women. Their mental wellbeing suffers, their relationships suffer and invariably their careers suffer too. I was totally unprepared for the aftermath of my surgical menopause and I'd like to ensure other women don't follow the same path. There has to be a better way. Many of the issues raised in the forthcoming pages are not solely relevant to surgical menopause, they will be equally applicable to menopause, irrespective of its individual nature.

Various commonalities came to the fore as I read through each woman's chapter. The anxiety surrounding that first 'post-operative poop', the hunched stoop, the belly clutching, and the hairy car rides home from hospital. The crushing fatigue of recovery, persistent 'swelly-belly', and the highly individualised recovery trajectories. The worrying lack of after-care and feelings of isolation. The dawning realisation that whilst everything had changed, nothing had changed. And yet, something had fundamentally shifted within each of us on a level far deeper than merely having a selection of our internal organs removed.

The primary objective of this book was to collate the authentic voices of those with lived experience of surgical menopause. I wanted to hear what women had to say. It was that simple. Personally, I know that writing can be therapeutic. We heal when our stories are shared in safe spaces. Some accounts focus specifically on the events that led up to surgery, some focus on the surgery itself, whilst others are primarily concerned with life after surgery. Many of us didn't give much thought to what our lives would look like when we left hospital. The prospect of being pain-free trumped everything else and we had our eyes firmly on the future.

As more and more women contributed, it occurred to me that many of the narratives held a richer significance. The narratives gave a glimpse into not just the state of women's hormonal healthcare, but also more importantly, they highlighted the sheer determination and tenacity of women to keep going. I feel deeply honoured and privileged to have read their stories. They are written with heart, and they demonstrate a courageous willingness to embrace vulnerability and to do so in a very public way.

I've been asked about the significance of the mountains on the cover. I purposefully chose mountains partly to represent the enormous personal treks each and every one of us in this book have undertaken. In 2020, I connected with an incredible woman from Galway, Ireland. That woman was Rachel Gotto. Rachel introduced me to a quote that I scribbled on a piece of paper at the time, and it has remained on my desk ever since – *"Give me mountains, I will climb them"*.

All contributors to this book are climbers, they are overcomers, and they are warriors. The majority fought before surgery, many for decades, and some are still fighting now. The battles are physical as well as emotional and psychological.

The mountains are also an indulgence on my part, in recognition of the stunningly beautiful & mountainous part of the world that I love and call my home, Scotland.

This book is not designed to alarm or deter you. My hope is that it might help inform you. To perhaps enable you to be better prepared if you're currently facing surgery that will put you into menopause. I feel passionately about raising awareness, because to quote Dr Peter Levine "without awareness, we have no choice". In the immediate aftermath of my surgery, I was numb and bewildered. I couldn't understand why I wasn't bouncing back. I felt alone and lost. However, I now know I was very far from alone in my experiences.

In addition to awareness, timely and appropriate intervention are key. I learnt the hard way that by not dealing with my issues as they arose, I added layer upon layer of complexity to what was already a complicated milieu of symptomology.

More often than not, we know our own bodies best, and if something doesn't feel right for you, follow it up as soon as you are able. As well as looking to professionals for help and advice, we also need to be prepared to advocate for ourselves and to look after ourselves as best as we possibly can. And I know that's often easier said than done, but we all have to start somewhere.

Please don't be tempted to use the personal stories as benchmarks for your own recovery though. Every single person will heal and recover differently, and very obviously the path of healing from laparoscopic surgery will be inherently different to healing after surgery involving an open abdominal incision.

In addition to featuring the voices of lived experience from a patient's perspective, for balance, I wanted to include viewpoints from folk working on the frontline of menopause care in the United Kingdom. Section 1 features contributions from both a menopause specialist doctor and a menopause specialist nurse. I need to add that none of the material in this book is intended as medical advice. For medical advice, it is imperative that you speak to your healthcare provider.

The 12 stories featured in section 2, are a reflection of the tremendous generosity of spirit that exists within the community of sisterhood. I am continually humbled by the willingness of women to share their experiences with the sole purpose of helping others avoid some of the pitfalls they themselves encountered. There is a huge depth of talent, creativity, wisdom, humour, compassion and strength within this community. It is testament to the fact that we are not in retreat. Far from it in fact.

The third and final section of this book very briefly introduces a few techniques that women featured in Chapters 1 to 12 have tried and found helpful. Clearly this section is not exhaustive. It's merely a snapshot of but a handful of available therapies out there, most of which incidentally have as their core aim, the reduction of stress. There is a message in there for all of us.

Helen Kemp
January 2021

Section One

Viewpoints

Dr Jane Davis MBChB, MRCGP, DRCOG, DFSRH, FHEA
Menopause Specialist and GP

Early on in my medical training, I knew my "why" was to advocate for women. Twenty years on I know that the key to gender equality is in providing excellent women's healthcare.

I work in Cornwall as a menopause specialist, GP, and contraception doctor. In every clinic, I am reminded of the importance of standing up for those going through the menopause. Amongst the most heart-breaking stories are those who have suffered poor management around surgical menopause. I was delighted, therefore, when Helen invited me to write for this ground-breaking book and hope that I can help by giving you a flavour of what it is like on the medical frontline, how if you are one of these women, you are very much not alone.

In May 2019, with the support of BBC Breakfast TV, some colleagues and I launched a social media campaign called *Rock My Menopause*[1]. We "#menovists" aim to support those going through the menopause and to smash its associated taboos. For support, advice, and some fun, please head to the Rock My Menopause[2] website and join the conversation.

Surgical menopause and informed consent

We know that surgical menopause is the term used to describe what happens when a woman has her ovaries removed. The ovaries, like the testicles are the sex hormone powerhouses of the body. Consider this scenario, which would never happen: "Shall we whip them out anyway?" said the surgeon as he swept into the anaesthetic room. John was lost for words; this was the first he had heard of the plan to remove his balls ....

When I first started training in menopause, I was incredulous that women could have their ovaries taken away without really understanding the consequences of what would happen to them. Imagine taking a man's testicles without them having any prior knowledge?

Why then do I still hear women tell me that they had similar experiences to this? They tell me that they did not feel in full control of the decision to remove their ovaries. They do not feel that they had a chance to think through the consequences of having their ovaries removed.

Approximately 4000 women in the UK undergo this operation each year. Removal of the ovaries, or "oophorectomy" is performed for several reasons. Many of these are potentially lifesaving such as treating cancer of the ovary or for preventing breast cancer in those with specific genetic mutations. For others, removal of the ovaries is a last resort in the battle against endometriosis or severe premenstrual dysphoric disorder (PMDD). However, we know for so many, this is life changing surgery.

I want to be clear here, I am not saying that you should not have surgery or should not have had it, I am saying that removal of the ovaries should never be agreed to without fully informed consent. I would also note that things have improved in the last few years, but we still have a long way to go. No woman should ever feel that she did not understand what was happening to her.

As doctors, we follow guidance from the General Medical Council[3]. For true informed consent, the guidance explains, a woman needs be given an opportunity to express what matters to her, to be given relevant information about the benefits and harms of proposed options and to be offered reasonable alternatives, including the option to take no action.

The impact of surgical menopause - what I see as a doctor

I see effects of surgical menopause compared to natural menopause like crash landing a plane in a desert rather than a turbulent, but controlled descent to the runway. Removal of the ovaries causes a sudden and complete loss of ovarian hormones. Even after natural menopause, the ovaries produce small amounts of these hormones. Therefore, the effect is felt more profoundly without treatment.

"I just don't feel like me".

This is one of the most common phrases that I hear after surgical menopause. Although it is saddening, it is not at all surprising. The female hormones, oestrogen, progesterone, and most of a woman's testosterone are produced in the ovary. When the ovaries are removed, the hormones levels plummet rapidly. The body and brain go "cold turkey". There are hormone receptors around our whole bodies. Female hormone withdrawal symptoms include, as we all know, hot flushes, insomnia, joint aches, and palpitations.

What I hear in clinic is women telling me that if it were just the physical stuff, they would perhaps cope, it is the emotional change, the mood swings, and the shift in their very being that is unbearable. This is because the brain is also withdrawing from the hormones normally produced by the ovary. The brain has been steeped in these hormones since puberty, it is no wonder that suddenly losing them causes a loss of sense of self.

Additionally, the hormone, testosterone gives the "vra vra vroom", and a dip in levels can cause the loss of sex drive. The get up and go tends to have got up and gone. The consequences can be devastating for relationships, work, and happiness. Although the adrenal glands continue to produce a little testosterone, the ovaries were the main testosterone factories. Sex drive can go completely "like a light being switched off". Along with extreme tiredness, often comes a loss of joy or even depression. Altogether, this is what seems to embody the sense of "I just don't feel like me anymore".

This can come on very suddenly or after a few weeks. Some women, I notice seem to be carried through by the adrenaline and shock of the surgery initially, followed by a crash, a physical and emotional crash a few weeks later.

Others are put on HRT immediately and come to see me months or years later to have the HRT adjusted. Remember, finding the right HRT is a bit like finding the right pair of shoes. You sometimes need to try a few before you find what suits you and your lifestyle best.

What is the long-term outlook after surgical menopause?

The psychological impact of losing the ovaries can be high for many women. Books like this give a wonderful insight into how this impact often plays out. I find women are culturally so incredibly stoical. We accept so much about our health as a "woman's lot". This is not just something you have to put up with, you can seek help and support and that is why it is wonderful to see books like this written.

Regarding the long-term effects of surgical menopause. It is very clear from scientific evidence that the ovaries provide a woman with long term protection of their heart, bones and probably of her brain too. Women going through menopause before the average age of 51 years should be offered some form of hormone replacement unless here is a reason that it is unsafe for them to take it. If you are interested, you will find this in the NICE guidance on Menopause Management[4].

Between 50 and 60, in the absence of other risk factors the benefits are likely to outweigh the risks for those who wish to take HRT for symptom relief. If you would like to know more, check out information on Rock My Menopause called: *HRT in a nutshell*.[5]

The use of HRT needs a full discussion with a clinician who knows how to make a full benefit and risk analysis. There is no arbitrary cut off for the age that a woman can use HRT if an annual review is made. Here you can discuss whether the benefits still outweigh the risks for you and plan for the year ahead.

Information -

"Women who are likely to go through menopause because of medical or surgical treatment are given information about menopause and fertility before they have their treatment" - Menopause Quality Standard [QS143], published 09 February 2017[6]

This is one of the five quality statements enshrined by NICE. For those of you who do not know, the National Institute of Clinical Excellence provides the clinical standards that we medics seek to reach in practice. NICE gives us direction in our clinical day a bit like using a GPS in the mist. I was fortunate enough to work on these guidelines back in 2017, with Linda Parkinson Hardman[7] from the Hysterectomy Association. Linda did a brilliant job of getting "information" on the agenda. Since then, I am pleased to see information has improved but we still have a long way to go.

I signpost women to Rock My Menopause[2], Women's Health Concern[8] and The Hysterectomy Association[7]. The Primary Care Women's Health Forum[9] work hard at supporting primary care practitioners to support women in the community, and they have a great website with bags of helpful information.

For younger women, the Daisy Network[10] provides excellent support for those who have undergone surgical menopause under the age of 40. I have been pleased to see that several trusts are producing specific information leaflets. However, the key to information is producing it in a way that makes most sense to that woman. This involves connecting with what matters to them and putting this is a language and format that works. Cultural sensitivity is essential; therefore, the best information comes when women support each other within communities. I love to see women supporting each other online, in support groups or over a coffee. However, it is important that there is a strong factual medical background, and that each woman can take this information to her clinician to help her work out how to individualise it for her.

So, there is loads more work to do here. Starting with this book. I would like to see more podcasts, videos and face to face workshops taking place. Watch this space for the advent of "group consultations" or "shared medical appointments". These are group medical appointments facilitated by a clinician. The research looks really promising for finding this a very supportive way of getting the information and support needed. This may not be everyone's cup of tea but with so few menopause specialists and a broke NHS, there is a lot of potential in the idea.

The root is education for the professionals. As a menopause trainer I can tell you the good news is that there is an enormous appetite for training amongst GP's. Each year more GP's and nurses are being trained to deliver excellent menopause care. Nurses are in a brilliant position to connect with women regarding menopause. Hazel Hayden is an inspirational nurse who has contributed to this book and Kath Abernethy was the first nurse to be chair of the British Menopause Society[11]. The Royal College of Nursing[12] are working hard on improving menopause education.

What advice would I give to a woman contemplating surgery?

As Helen says earlier in the introduction, forewarned is forearmed. Do your research, ask other women about their experiences. Book a specific appointment with your doctor to go through the risks and benefits that are relevant to you. Know if you are going to go for HRT and ensure you have your prescription ready to go after surgery, your anaesthetist will be able to tell you when you can start it.

HRT, why is it important?

HRT as we have touched on above protects the heart, bones and probably the brain long term. Having treated women for years I know that no medicine is as good as HRT at controlling menopause symptoms. There are alternatives if you cannot take it or do not wish to do so, however.

Do not forget vaginal health. The vagina and bladder are greedy for oestrogen. Plummeting oestrogen levels may well cause vaginal dryness, itching, pricking and pain with intercourse. Sometimes this is accompanied by needing to wee more or finding you have less bladder control. The good news is that vaginal oestrogens are generally well tolerated and there are very few women for whom it is unsuitable.

What about testosterone?

In my experience, women who have had their ovaries removed, can often need testosterone to get them feeling balanced again. Most significantly this tends to be if the sexual desire has gone. Also, women can feel excessively tired, achy, and low when they are testosterone deficient. This makes sense as the greatest proportion of testosterone is made in the ovaries. There is still a little from the adrenal glands, but it is not usually enough to make people feel "like them".

The use of testosterone is mentioned in the NICE guidance as worth considering for low sexual desire if HRT alone does not help. However, many GP's will feel unsure about prescribing it. This is because there is no licence in the UK for women to use testosterone. To help, there are some great practical tips for prescribers from the Primary Care Women's Health Forum[13]

The key is to get the oestrogen right first, then to take bloods. Without getting too technical, the bloods are very specific, looking at how much of the testosterone the body can actually "see". Once a baseline level is established as low, then a trial of testosterone may be considered.

In the UK we have testosterone designed for use in males, usually in the form of a sachet called Testogel, which you need to make last 10 days. It is applied to the skin usually the thighs, bloods are taken after 8 weeks or so to check if the levels are still within a normal physiological range for a woman. If there has been no improvement, then it can be stopped. If all is well then it is a good idea to keep an eye on these bloods and review regularly.

In recent years we have started importing a testosterone from Australia which is tested for use in females. This is called "Androfeme1" - you can look it up online. This is only available privately and not licensed in the UK. I like using this product as it is reassuring that it has been licensed for women in Australia. I would like to see it available in mainstream UK, particularly for women who have had their ovaries removed.

I do not want you to think that testosterone is the panacea for all ills. It will not make you feel 21 again or guarantee that you and your partner will enjoy mind blowing sex. However, in my experience, testosterone can make a huge difference to women after removal of the ovaries. It is worth some serious consideration if you feel that you may benefit from it.

The Menopause Landscape - what is on the horizon?

There are "ripples being made, waves will form, tsunamis will come..." Dr Nighat Arif GP, BBC Breakfast "Wake up to the Menopause" May 2019 [14]

Today, there is undoubtedly a groundswell of opinion demanding better menopause care. This is from women themselves but also, clinicians, activists, and politicians. More women are knowing and saying what they want. The medical profession is feeling more confident in menopause management as training improves. As a medical school tutor, I can tell you that students are well informed about menopause. It now features in the school curriculum in England, thanks to the work of campaigns such as "#MakeMenopauseMatter".

The All-Party Parliamentary Group on Women's Health[15] "has our back aiming to empower women to ensure that they can make an informed choice about the best treatment for them and that they are treated with dignity and respect".

They are working hard with clinicians and patients raise awareness nationally about conditions such as surgical menopause.

The future is bright for menopause care, but for many of you there may be a long journey ahead to recovery. I ask you firstly find what you need to do take care of yourselves. When you are strong you can help others. Please keep supporting each other rattling cages for improved information and care around surgical menopause.

Finally, do not forget to keep standing up for each other and keep smashing those taboos. Let's help the next set of women to go through surgical menopause to have the best experience that they can and live a happier fuller life, as a result.

Dr Jane Davis works in Cornwall as a menopause specialist, GP, and contraception doctor. Jane holds the FSRH Advanced Certificate in Menopause Care and is recognised by the British Menopause Society as a specialist in her field. A feminist writer and medical editor for Her Life Her Health magazine, you can find Dr Davis at work on https://stermemedical.uk/ or on Twitter @DrJaneDavis1

[1]*Rock My Menopause on BBC Breakfast TV: www.youtube.com/watch?v=PdAPBhCFYAE*

[2]*https://rockmymenopause.com*

[3]*https://www.gmc-uk.org/-/media/documents/gmc-guidance-for-doctors---decision-making-and-consent-english_pdf-84191055.pdf?la=en&hash=BE327A1C584627D12BC51F66E790443F0E0651DA see also "Informed Consent and the Revised GMC Guidance." Medical Solicitors, 26 Nov. 2020, http://www.medical-solicitors.com/informed-consent-and-the-revised-gmc-guidance*

[4]*"Overview | Menopause: Diagnosis and Management | Guidance | NICE." Nice.org.Uk, NICE, 12 Nov. 2015, www.nice.org.uk/guidance/ng23.*

[5]*Davis, Jane. "HRT in a Nutshell." Rock My Menopause, www.rockmymenopause.com/portfolio-item/hrt-in-a-nutshell*

[6]*https://www.nice.org.uk/guidance/qs143*

[7]*https://healthyhappywoman.co.uk/hysterectomy-information/what-is-a-hysterectomy/*

[8]*https://www.womens-health-concern.org*

[9]*https://pcwhf.co.uk*

[10]*https://www.daisynetwork.org*

[11]*https://thebms.org.uk*

[12]*https://www.rcn.org.uk*

[13]PCWHF. *"10 Top Tips on Testosterone Use for Women."* Primary Care Women's Health Forum, https://pcwhf.co.uk/resources/10-top-tips-on-testosterone-use-for-women

[14]*"BBC One - Breakfast, Dr Nighat Arif Talks about Menopause and Working with BAME Women."* BBC, 13 May 2019, www.bbc.co.uk/programmes/p0792jx6

[15]*All-Party Parliamentary Group on Women's Health,* www.appgwomenshealth.org/about#about-the-group.

Hazel Hayden MSc, RN, ANP
Menopause Nurse Specialist

I had been seeing a patient, primarily to manage her contraception as a means of stopping menorrhagia (heavy bleeding) and fibroids. Eventually this woman had a hysterectomy which included the removal of both ovaries, and she went into acute menopause. The gynaecologist who had been treating her (and who performed the surgery) had not warned her that would happen. That was the first time in my professional life that I came across surgical menopause.

I went from being a nurse who looked after and knew how to manage menopause well, to a nurse who had to do lots of research into surgical menopause! It was a huge shock to me that this could happen. I endeavored to find out as much as I could to help this woman. She had gone from someone who could manage on Evorel Sequi to being symptomatic on Evorel 100.

That woman worked as an accountant running her own company and she suddenly felt the ground beneath her fall away. I felt completely out of my depth. I had never been in this situation before. I read information from the British Menopause Society, and I had to dig deeper. It ended up being a long slow process with this woman coming to see me monthly until eventually we managed to get her back on an even keel. Although looking back now, not as well as I could have done.

So, that was the start of my story of working with women in surgical menopause, and that was 7 years ago. Before that, I had managed 8 years without knowingly seeing a woman with a surgical menopause, presumably because they were seeing their GP for symptom management. This shook my belief in my ability. As a result, I became more and more interested in the effects of surgical menopause on a woman's mental as well as physical health.

The term 'surgical menopause' refers to an induced menopause as a result of the removal of both ovaries (bilateral oophorectomy) before the age of 45 or natural menopause. A hysterectomy involves the removal of the uterus, which can be performed laparoscopically, vaginally, or via an abdominal incision. Typical reasons for undergoing a hysterectomy (with or without removal of one or both ovaries) may include endometriosis and/or adenomyosis, both of which are very painful conditions. But women who have an inherited risk of cancer may elect to have surgery to reduce their risk of later developing cancer.

Women undergoing a bilateral oophorectomy go into instant menopause and can have severe symptoms. They are at an increased risk of osteoporosis, cardiovascular disease, sexual dysfunction and may well need counselling around loss of fertility. These women will need hormone replacement therapy (HRT) and also testosterone. Very often, these women are not informed about the effects their surgery will have on their bodies or their lives. Therefore, the symptoms of surgical menopause are usually distressing and difficult to cope with.

For women who have had a hysterectomy due to endometriosis it is important that they are given a combined oestrogen and progesterone form of HRT for a few years. This is because although most of the endometriosis will have been removed, there may well be one microscopic patch left that oestrogen may well reactivate. This residual endometriosis could potentially change into a malignancy many years later. However, at the average natural age of menopause (51), the progesterone should be stopped to ensure there is no increased risk of breast cancer.

There are positive effects of surgical menopause, including a reduced risk of ovarian cancer in women who have an increased inherited risk of ovarian cancer. For some women it can also decrease their risk of breast cancer. It also reduces the pain of endometriosis in the pelvic area, as well as reducing the risk of ovarian pain due to endometriosis adhesions in the area.

In practice, the main issue I encounter with women in surgical menopause seems to be a reduction in their sense of joy in life, plus the rollercoaster of having to manage their menopausal symptoms, often at a young age. When I see these women in my clinic (and they are usually below the age of 40), the main issues they typically present with are:

- Hot flushes
- Joint and muscle aches
- Low mood
- Loss of libido
- Anxiety
- Vaginal dryness and pain when having intercourse

It is a fine balancing act to try and stabilise the hormones in order to reduce each woman's symptoms. I call it a jigsaw puzzle where all the key ingredients need to be in perfect balance, and this balance can easily go haywire. This is due in part to the effect of testosterone.

As young women, testosterone is our dominant hormone. It is produced in the ovaries and a small amount comes from the adrenal glands. It gives women their get up and go, confidence and libido. As a result of surgical menopause, there will be very little testosterone in the body, as well as barely any oestrogen. The body will crave oestrogen, and metabolise any residual testosterone into oestrogen, leaving almost no testosterone.

HRT for younger women may well need to be at higher doses and in this situation, it is worth getting oestrogen (oestradiol) levels checked. There is a form of HRT called Tibolone which is not oestrogen or progesterone, but it provides an oestrogenic, progestrogenic and androgenic effect which can help particularly in older women. However, for younger women it does not provide enough oestrogen to reduce all their symptoms.

Sadly, in the United Kingdom, testosterone is not licensed and is therefore only available privately or if you see a specialist menopause practitioner. If a practice has a person who specialises in menopause they may well be happy to give testosterone on a private prescription. Testosterone is a gel that is applied to the skin daily.

In clinic, it is often a case of trial and error to get all the hormones balanced, however it is important to try it all for at least 2 months.

There are also lifestyle factors to consider:

- Regular exercise - weight bearing to protect bones
- Weight management - keep BMI under 30 as this lowers the risk of cancer
- Cognitive Behavioural Therapy - can help with some symptoms such as hot flushes
- Diet - reduce sugar and alcohol. This can reduce night sweats and may also help with mood.
- Think about Vitamin D supplementation, this can help with bones.

The biggest issue encountered around surgical menopause is a lack of knowledge of Healthcare Professionals and the women who undergo the surgery and this needs to be changed. We need more menopause trained HCPs at all levels and we need women to have better access to education.

Hazel has been managing women's health in GP surgeries for 15 years, and now runs her own private menopause clinic in Bristol. Hazel holds an MSc in Sexual Health in Menopause, a British Menopause Society Certificate in Menopause, a Women's Health Practitioner Diploma and a Diploma in Nutrition. Find Hazel at: www.bristolmenopause.com

Section Two

Stories from women in surgical menopause

Chapter One

Karen Kenning, 51

My favourite author, Amanda Prowse, always has me hooked by the end of the first chapter of every book she writes. She's an incredibly talented writer, with a style based in real life and characters that you easily warm to and accept. She tells stories everyone can relate to. She has the ability to make you believe and accept what she's telling you.

With the benefit of hindsight, the trouble I have with my own story, is that I now feel somewhat detached from it. It's hard to look back and remember how bad things got. Now that I feel well and healthy, it feels very much as if what I'm about to share with you happened to somebody else.

The introduction is an important part of any story – where you learn a bit about the characters, set the scene, and consciously or otherwise, decide whether your interest has been piqued enough to go on to read more. A lot hinges on the first few lines of each story, and it's important to get it right. I'd like to tell you about my journey.

I use the "j" word deliberately. Strictly Come Dancing is my guilty pleasure for sure. Strictly on the TV means winter nights, woolly socks and jumpers and the run up to Christmas. It's cosy, it's familiar and it's something guaranteed to always cheer me up. I watch everyone twirling around on the dance floor and I admire their efforts knowing that the closest I'll ever get to taking part from anywhere except my sofa, is borrowing this word that we hear so many times in every series. If you look at the definition of the word, "a long and often difficult process of personal change and development", then I can justify said word and, in the right context, embrace it as an almost perfect way to describe my story! Interestingly, as I write this, I realised that Strictly Come Dancing came to our screens 17 years ago – and that's still slightly less time than I've been dealing with menopause symptoms. That's not designed to scare you off at all. It's simply a detail that's relevant.

I find talking about myself to be the most difficult and excruciating thing. I'm sure that a lot of people do. Ask me about my family though and I'll happily comply!

I could wax lyrical for hours about my amazing, handsome husband who works so hard to support our family. I could tell you how hard I've found lockdown without my strongest support and best friend by my side, and how being in different countries during a pandemic has been stressful and exhausting. I could tell you about my kind and thoughtful boys (who, as much as I adore the very bones of them, have pushed me to the limits and beyond during lockdown). I could also tell you about my beautiful puppies and describe their character traits in the greatest amount of detail and with joyful disregard for your boredom threshold and show you endless adorable photos of these most photogenic beasties.

I'll spare you all of that and simply say that I'm a very happily married mum of 2 young adults, living in the beautiful North East part of Scotland with my doggy squad, some guinea pigs and soon I'll be adding a clutch of hens. My life is fairly unassuming. I class myself as incredibly lucky that I get to spend lots of time in our beautiful garden which I enjoy immensely, and my life centres around my wonderful husband, my sons and my animals. I am healthy. I am happy. I am loved. And now, finally, I am back to full health and fortunate in so many ways.

When I was asked to contribute to this book, I immediately said yes. I was thrilled that the subject of menopause, and specifically surgical menopause, was being written about at all, and that it was being tackled in an open, honest and hopefully helpful way by women who have experienced it. How I wish there had been something for me to read before I started down the path that my early hysterectomy took me. I don't know whether it would have changed the outcome for me, but perhaps it would have helped me to solve my menopause riddle far quicker.

I was also embarrassed to have been asked. Not because I have any issue talking about all things menopause, but I do feel completely and utterly ashamed and unsure whether I am ready to share my experience again. Because in sharing, you have to delve deep and recall some of the very things that you've worked so hard to repair and move on from. So, the real reason for sharing, for me at least, is to help even one other woman understand that what's happening to her is real, not imagined, and can be helped, and to give her the courage to advocate for herself.

I'm nothing special. In as much as anyone is, I'm pretty average. I don't say that to in any way demean or diminish myself. I'm simply pointing out that I could be any woman. That's so important. Menopause will happen to every woman. It's an entirely natural part of a woman's life. Each woman will experience it differently. My life, my experiences and the choices I've made along the way are no better and no worse than anyone else's. None of what I will describe is a bid for sympathy, an attempt to suggest that I've had a tougher time than anyone else, nor is it a "poor me" story. This is simply what happened to me.

When my youngest son was 9 months old, as a result of continuous bleeding prior to, during my pregnancy and after the birth, I was told I needed a hysterectomy. I don't remember any great, lengthy discussions. I don't remember any exhaustive measures to investigate the issues I'd been having, and, at that point, I don't think that I looked any further forward than getting the situation I found myself in remedied. I'd tried options like the Mirena coil and various contraceptive pills. The doctors couldn't tell me what was specifically wrong, and indeed, there seemed to be nothing particularly wrong – no fibroids, no reason for what was happening to me, except that I never got much of a break from the continual bleeding. As a young mum with 2 small children, I was continually exhausted and needed some relief.

I'd always had gynae problems and had two extremely difficult pregnancies with both myself and my babies in danger. I was sad that I'd be unable to have any more children, I didn't feel as if my family was complete, but I knew that I'd barely made it through each pregnancy, and it would have been foolish to attempt another. At that point, I counted myself lucky for the two beautiful boys that I had, and resigned myself to the news – I think what I actually mean, is that I did what I was told.

Looking back, I think there was almost certainly an element for me, of wanting to be done with doctors. I had spent the last 4 months of my second pregnancy in a hospital bed under constant supervision, with both my life and the life of my unborn baby in jeopardy because of placenta previa. I was embarrassed that it felt to me as if my body was constantly letting me down. I didn't understand why other women seemed to have normal periods or easy pregnancies whilst my periods had always been for 3 weeks out of 4 since my early teens.

I continued to bleed all the way through both pregnancies, and following the birth of my son, the bleeding became a constant. I was exhausted, but this was my "normal" and had been for a long time, and up till that point it hadn't really impacted on anyone except for me. I couldn't understand what was happening and all I wanted was to be fit and healthy in order to look after my babies. I had such high expectations that the hysterectomy was going to be the answer to all my problems.

The surgery went ahead. I was 34 years old, and post op, I was sent on my way with little more information than I shouldn't lift anything for 6 weeks, refrain from sex for the same amount of time and that, because I'd retained my ovaries, I would go into menopause "at the normal time". I didn't know then what the normal time was, and it didn't occur to me to ask. The very little I knew about menopause told me it was way off sometime in the future, and nothing for me to worry about at that particular point! I was focused only on getting home to a more normal life; a life with no more bleeding and the energy to look after and enjoy my gorgeous little boys.

I had such high hopes for the improvement this major surgery would bring to my life. Except, despite the hysterectomy, I was shocked and scared to find that my periods continued. I wondered if I was imagining the appearance of the usual monthly bleed and I had to convince myself to go back to my GP once again. Far from being done with doctors, things took a frightening turn for me.

It didn't cross my mind that periods after a hysterectomy was something that could happen. From the "high" and expectation that the bleeding of my past would be gone, I was suddenly thrown into the depths of despair, facing all sorts of terrifying cancer related scenarios, and as a young mum, with two small children to consider, my fear about what was happening to me was enormous. I even started making plans in my head for what would happen to my children if I was no longer around.

When I summoned up the courage to make an appointment, my GP was very blunt, and told me not to be "ridiculous". He needlessly pointed out that I'd had a hysterectomy. I found his reaction upsetting and unhelpful, and it did nothing to alleviate my fears. Although I understood his confusion, even though I had the evidence myself, I didn't really believe or understand what was happening either. My appointment left me feeling frightened and confused with no idea what was wrong.

I looked elsewhere for help. An email to the British Menopause Society to explain my circumstances baffled them too, and it was a further two to three years, and a posting to Germany before a gynaecologist there was able to work out what was wrong. After an excruciatingly worrying time, keyhole surgery was done to correct the issue. This involved removing the last part of my cervix. My previous C-section surgery had left some scarring, and unbeknown to me, a portion of my cervix had become scarred to my bladder. The surgeon had chosen to leave this behind during my hysterectomy rather than risk any issues or damage to my bladder. The problem was diagnosed quickly and corrected without issue by my German gynaecologist. Finally, the bleeding stopped.

To my mind, this piece of great news should have brought an end to my health issues, but to add to the difficulties I experienced, within weeks of my hysterectomy, I begun to experience symptoms that I now recognise as menopause related. I pushed all of these things to the back of my mind to begin with, sure that the anxiety from continual unexplained bleeding was having an impact on my mind as well as the rest of my body.

The symptoms were many, varied, and relentless though and added to the general feeling of despair and unhappiness that I felt. Given the reaction from my GP when I told him about my post-op bleeding, I had a reluctance to add anything else into the mix. I didn't want to be a nuisance, and I didn't want to feel like a fool again.

It took an enormous amount of effort every time I convinced myself it was time to consult a GP again.

I put up with hot flushes so severe I would be left embarrassingly drenched. Low mood that would come out of nowhere and disappear again as fast as it appeared. Insomnia so debilitating that I struggled by on 2-3 hours' sleep each night. Fatigue. Sore joints. Heart palpitations. Brain fog. Dizziness. Headaches. I didn't know what was happening to me, and more worryingly, the doctors I went to see didn't either.

There was always an explanation for each symptom, but never a look at the symptoms as a package. The sweats were because we lived in Riyadh, even when I argued that I kept my home air conditioning set to Glasgow temperatures! When the flushes continued in Germany, I was treated for hyperhidrosis. Everything dried up except the flushes! The insomnia was because I had two small children – and nobody gets much sleep when they have small children. The symptoms in general, were seen as an anxious reaction to the unexpected health issues I'd experienced, but even after the period issue was resolved, symptoms remained. Every symptom had a seemingly reasonable explanation – and coupled with my previous poor experience with my GP, I didn't know enough about menopause to enable me to recognise what was happening myself and argue my case. I always accepted what I was told.

The symptoms impacted every aspect of my life – at home, in the workplace, with family and relationships. Life was a constant struggle. Countless trips to various GPs continued, and finally, 9 years after my hysterectomy, a lady GP finally made the suggestion that I may be experiencing symptoms of the menopause.

Blood tests didn't support this theory, although we now know these can be unreliable due to fluctuating hormone levels, and a discussion about HRT as an option to help regardless of the blood test results was dismissed, because I have always suffered with migraines. My lack of knowledge, and my assumption that GP's know more than their patients, stopped me from debating this any further, and, disappointed that there was nothing medical to help me, at least I finally had a likely explanation for the catalogue of symptoms that had plagued me for such a long time.

Since my GP couldn't help me, I took to the internet and spent hours looking for answers to the endless symptoms. My nights were spent trying not to spontaneously combust over and over again, in a room that even my dogs sometimes refused to sleep in. The windows were always wide open even in the depths of a Scottish winter, the temperature as low as I could possibly get it and there were gale force winds blowing not just from the windows, but from a permanent fan in the corner of the room.

I had a meditation track playing constantly in the background. If I didn't have it playing, I couldn't get to sleep, but when the track finished, that would wake me up again - but not playing it meant I didn't fall asleep in the first place. It became a vicious circle, and the lack of sleep and how to fix it, all consuming. I played the hokey-cokey endlessly, with one leg in and one leg out of the covers in a desperate bid to cool off until it became all too apparent that there wouldn't be any sleep again, and I would shift to the living room to finish the night there.

Days were spent trying to ignore the overwhelming fatigue caused by the night-time shenanigans and simply get on with the job of putting one foot in front of the other. I hadn't had a period in 17 years, yet I got period pain. From a phantom uterus? Everything was dry: my skin, my nails, my hair, my eyes, my vagina, my sense of humour! I got anxious because I was tired, and my hormone levels were all over the place. When I'm tired and stressed, I get migraines. I was always tired and stressed, so the migraines were incessant.

Some days there was an overwhelming sadness that came out of nowhere and it was just such a slog to do anything. Don't even talk to me about the tears. The Six O'clock News – the daftest story could bring me to tears. MasterChef for goodness sake! More crying. School parents' nights – sobs! It was like a tap I had no control over!

The lack of help from my GP meant that I was left desperately floundering about trying to find something that worked. I definitely felt as if I was on my own. I was so fed up with feeling awful. It wasn't something I talked about with friends, family members or work colleagues. I was sick and tired of feeling the way that I did, and I didn't feel that I should share my misery with the people around me. My symptoms had been going on for years, and GPs never gave me anything that helped, so therefore, was there really even anything wrong with me, except being a monumental moan? No. I didn't want to share that with anyone. It was lonely. I was so unhappy, and life wasn't fun.

There was nobody talking about the menopause. Do you remember when you became a teenager, about to hit puberty, start periods, find out about sex? There seemed to be a wealth of knowledge then. Books and pamphlets handed out, talks at school, information from your friends, your mother, magazines, everyone falling over themselves to give you more information than you'd ever need. The same a few years later when you find yourself pregnant. Suddenly as much information as you could ever want is raining down on you from doctors, midwifes, health visitors and every woman who's ever been pregnant. So why does it all stop when we get to the menopause stage?

The fact that there is nothing out there, means that you get your information from the internet and the internet becomes your non-judgemental friend who knows everything. It tells you that you need black cohosh, and sage. Red clover, and mung beans. Magnesium drinks, magnesium capsules, even magnesium rubs for aching bones and joints. Cooling pillows and scarves. Bamboo vests and knickers. Whisper-quiet fans that won't disturb your sleep. Magnets for your knickers, magnets for your wrists. Sprays for your pillows, cream for your temples. Fitness trackers to record just how much sleep you're not having, and to taunt you with your recommended 7 hours a night. Shampoo to restructure your dry, menopausal hair. Creams to nourish your dry, menopausal hands. Gels and pessaries to nourish your dry and tired vagina.

I know there's more! I have bought more. I know I have. And some things have been more successful than others. There are lots of options for desperate menopausal woman to spend money on, and in my misery, I tried a significant number of them!

I struggled on for another 7 years. The trips to the GP continued. I felt more and more like the patient every doctor dreads. The "here we go again" woman. I felt eye rolls, even if I never quite saw them. I genuinely had to gather myself every time I made an appointment, resigned to the fact that I'd come away without a resolution once again. No amount of antidepressants helped. None of the migraine preventatives made a difference. Heart scans proved negative. Beta-blockers didn't help. It didn't matter which symptoms I went with; I couldn't seem to get a resolution and I always ended up more fed up, frustrated and disillusioned with each visit.

Despite being reasonably articulate, I felt that I simply must not be communicating the level of despair I felt, and after 16 years of debilitating and all-consuming symptoms, I was completely and utterly fed up with everything. I had no motivation. I wondered what the point was when life was so miserable. I'd spent the whole of my children's lives fighting and struggling with one symptom after another. There was a distinct lack of joy, and despite all my efforts, I just couldn't fix myself.

Frustrated and fed up, I began to search for answers once again. I found a Facebook group with women chatting and offering support to one another. It was refreshing. Women talking about menopause. I no longer felt alone. As a result of this group, the chance to work as a moderator on a new community forum came up. The forum was specifically to help women coping with menopause symptoms. It was the perfect opportunity for me and having access to ask the experts on the website all sorts of questions, I discovered that, despite what the GP had told me, HRT was an option for me in the form of transdermal patches or gel.

Armed with this new information, and desperate to feel better, I called my new GP. He was sympathetic, he was informed, and he listened. Best of all, he agreed that I could try the patches. He talked about the possible side effects, he discussed the risks and benefits, and I finally felt that I'd found a doctor who was informed about the treatment of menopause symptoms.

That prescription changed my life.

Two years on, with a few tweaks to the strength of prescription, and the addition of privately prescribed testosterone, I have my life back. All of the symptoms that I struggled so much with in previous years are kept in check by the HRT that I didn't know I needed. Ironically, when menopause was floated as a possible answer, the very thing that stopped me getting HRT were the migraines, which have significantly reduced with the use of oestrogen.

I'm frustrated that I wasn't better prepared for my operation. I wasn't aware that having my womb removed might shock my ovaries into failing. I wasn't warned about the signs and symptoms to look out for as a result. And, when I presented with those signs and symptoms to the very many GP's I saw over subsequent year, none of them picked up and made the connection between my hysterectomy and the symptoms I was experiencing. The very people that I went to for help, didn't know enough, if anything, about menopause.

Surgical menopause for me, was brutal – but, it didn't have to be, and that's the real shame of it. I look back and know that a lack of information was the kicker. I didn't know enough. My doctors didn't know enough. It's so heart breaking that it's really as low down and basic as that.

These days, I feel well. So well that it's strange to think how different my life has become. It's hard to look back and remember all of the struggles. I haven't described everything that happened to me. In the place I am now, it's hard to comprehend that I couldn't see what seems so obvious to me now, and I'm sad that my experience changed my personality and my confidence in myself in such a detrimental way. I look back and see a different woman. I wonder how I managed to keep going. How I managed to look after a family and keep a job. Relationships faltered. Friendships died.

I read stories on the very many menopause forums and groups now available. Some things don't seem to have changed at all. Women still struggle to find a GP with experience in menopause. They are still being offered inappropriate treatments and dismissed when they present with menopause symptoms. Other things have changed dramatically since I first started experiencing symptoms, with more evidence-based information available to help guide women to the help and treatments they need. It's a step in the right direction that enables women to advocate for themselves. But it's still far harder than it should have to be. GP's and other doctors still don't have the training they need in order to help properly, and there are still so many myths and old-fashioned ideas that need to be squashed.

I see stories from women feeling awful for months at a time before they got help in the form of HRT. I wonder why I was prepared to put up with feeling awful for all those years. And yet, I did what I could. I asked for help. Even when I felt that I was simply being a nuisance and a hypochondriac, I did keep going back for help, only to be dismissed.

I can only tell you, that when you feel awful, when you are so exhausted that your only thoughts are to get through the day as best and as quickly as you can, you simply don't have the reserves to keep fighting and do anything other than exist. When the people that you go to for help can't unravel the mystery for you either, and there's no one else that you can turn to for help, things become almost insurmountable.

Now that I feel well and healthy again, it's so much easier to advocate for myself. To ask questions and debate with my GP if I don't agree with something. For the longest time, I accepted things that I didn't have the energy to question, and I find that very sad indeed.

The solution for me is a little patch of oestrogen and a blob of testosterone gel. Something so simple that took such a long time to get, but which has transformed my life and my health.

The key to everything is information. Do your research. Find your reputable and knowledgeable sources and ask questions. Don't assume that your doctors will always know the answer, and don't be afraid of going elsewhere to find a solution if you don't get one from your doctor. Listen to your body. Track everything. Trust your instincts. Find your voice.

And know, that as hard as life can be, as awful as symptoms can get, with the right help, you really will feel well again.

Karen tweets as: @Karen_Kenning

Chapter Two

Sarah Williams, 49

Despite the loud and proud conversations I see in my social media echo chamber about menopause, there are still thousands of women who are not accessing reliable information about reproductive health. Many are living lives challenged by symptoms that could be easily treated, instead of holding them back from reaching their potential. This is down to a lack of awareness and education about all types of women's health conditions, including surgical menopause.

I'm often contacted by people looking for information and support in their surgical menopause journey and to date have had little choice in where to signpost for reading about the experiences of others in surgical menopause. I have purchased many menopause books expecting to see a chapter at least dedicated to surgical menopause only to be disappointed by only a fleeting reference to it. This book will go a huge way to filling the information gap about surgical menopause and I'm delighted to be contributing to it.

Around 1900, life expectancy was no more than 50 years of age. Now in Wales at least, we can expect to hang around a little longer, 84.3 years to be exact. So, we now have, hopefully, 30 years or more to live and function well in this state. For those of us in surgical menopause following a bilateral oophorectomy (the removal of both ovaries) we have to journey through this phase managing what is really a long-term health condition. Experiencing the sudden loss of certain hormones is no fun. It's *not* the same as a natural menopause and it's not called a 'cliff-edge menopause' for nothing.

It is important to give context to my arrival at surgical menopause. The condition I was experiencing is still not a mainstream topic and there is often misdiagnosis of it with more serious mental illness. This of course means that some people will be incorrectly medicated which can have implications for long term health. So, forgive my self-indulgence for a page or so but it's often by highlighting the authentic voice of lived experience that lightbulb moments occur. And sometimes, these can be pivotal in turning around someone's health and wellbeing.

So, rewind to 2012, aged 41, I attended a gynaecology appointment to investigate the possibility of fibroids. I was feeling low in mood and very tearful, thankfully this was picked up on. After talking with me about this and other symptoms that I was having difficulty with on a regular basis, my consultant recommended I tracked my daily mood and physical symptoms in case of the presence of 'severe PMS'. After just the first month or so of data capture, there was a clear difference in symptoms across the weeks.

After capturing 2 full menstrual cycles it was clear that I was experiencing shifts in my physical and psychological symptoms directly relating to the lead up to my period. For 2 weeks a month I was left with physical symptoms that were flooring me only to be swiftly relieved by the onset of my period. I had premenstrual dysphoric disorder (PMDD), a suspected hormone sensitivity disorder of the brain which sees a severe negative reaction to the natural rise and fall of oestrogen and progesterone.

This is not PMS that can be alleviated or managed with a good bar of Green & Blacks and a bubble bath. Undiagnosed and untreated PMDD destroys lives. It is currently estimated that 1 in 20, that's around 800,000 people in the UK have the condition and 30% of these will attempt suicide[1]. Onset and worsening of PMDD can be triggered by hormonal events such as menarche, pregnancy, peri-menopause. Tick! Tick! Tick! The final trigger of peri-menopause seeming to be for me the one that tipped me over the edge and saw me pleading for help, and to 'get it all out'.

According to the International Association of Pre-Menstrual Disorders (IAPMD) the symptoms of PMDD (5 of which must be present for a diagnosis with one of them being in the first four) are:

❖ Mood/emotional changes e.g., mood swings, feeling suddenly sad or tearful, or increased sensitivity to rejection
❖ Irritability, anger, or increased interpersonal conflict
❖ Depressed mood, feelings of hopelessness, feeling worthless or guilty
❖ Anxiety, tension, or feelings of being keyed up or on edge
❖ Decreased interest in usual activities e.g., work, school, friends, hobbies
❖ Difficulty concentrating, focusing, or thinking; brain fog
❖ Tiredness or low energy
❖ Changes in appetite, food cravings, overeating, or binge eating
❖ Hypersomnia (excessive sleepiness) or insomnia (trouble falling/staying asleep)
❖ Feeling overwhelmed or out of control
❖ Physical symptoms such as breast tenderness or swelling, joint or muscle pain, bloating or weight gain

This lifelong sensitivity to hormone fluctuations was becoming unbearable as the hormonal fluctuations in peri-menopause exacerbated my situation. Removal of my ovaries was becoming the only sensible option if I were to be able to enjoy a life where I could thrive and have any chance of reaching my potential.

However, before surgery for PMDD could be agreed, my consultant needed to be satisfied that this was the correct and only remaining course of action for me. I was trialled for a few months on a gonadotropin releasing hormone agonist (GnRHa) treatment which works by bringing on a temporary, reversible menopause, effectively 'switching off' the ovaries for a while and stopping your ovaries from producing hormones.

My menstrual periods stopped, and I entered a chemical menopause. Within a couple of months my anxiety had dissipated, moods become more stable and I noticed I was more easily able to work. I was having less disruption in my personal life and relationships. A review after 8 months resulted in the decision that I should have the hysterectomy. Cause for celebration, yes, but not without an emotional dip as I came to terms with not having any more birth children and what that might mean for my partner and I.

If you think you have PMDD, tell your GP and someone you trust. This ensures you have a shared problem and are not dealing with it alone. Use NAPS[2] and IAPMD[1] for their amazing resources. There are plenty of online support groups, one of which is a peer support group I set up to reach out to others in Wales affected by PMDD. It's called PMDD-Pod[3].

It's important to mention that during all of this time I was blissfully unaware of the existence of the phase of reproductive life that is 'peri-menopause' even though I had for some time been experiencing, and seeking help for, some of the symptoms. By my early 40's these are some of the symptoms I was experiencing:

❖ Electric shocks (I didn't seek help for this, I just thought it was odd)
❖ Palpitations
❖ Pins and needles
❖ Dry skin resulting in scratching my calves until they bled. On seeking help for this, one medic suggested I may need to "shave my legs more often"
❖ My beautiful conker brown shiny hair started to turn into wiry, coarse curls
❖ Worsening anxiety and panic attacks
❖ Tears, lots of tears!
❖ Concentration and focus issues
❖ Elbow & joint pain and swelling in my finger joints (I thought I had gout!)
❖ Bladder problems

❖ Increasing heavy menstrual bleeding, (I also had undiagnosed adenomyosis) my period lasted around 10 days and was littered with clots around 10cm diameter.

So, thankfully, on November 29th 2018, aged 47, I underwent a total abdominal hysterectomy with bilateral salpingo oophorectomy (TAH-BSO) at Nuffield Health, Vale Hospital in Hensol. I had been fortunate enough for my NHS waiting time to be approaching a time that would exceed the limit and so I was offloaded onto the Nuffield to experience the pleasure of a private room and more importantly, a 5-star menu choice. I was very well cared for by staff and was reluctant to leave!

Surgery has been life-changing for me. As my periods have permanently ceased, so have the fluctuations in my sex hormones. I will always have the hormone sensitivity however, and this has to be taken into consideration when planning my hormone replacement therapy (HRT).

I was all up for HRT having already started using addback oestrogen patches during the temporary chemical menopause as part of the treatment regime for PMDD. I'd also thoroughly researched the long-term health risks of surgical menopause associated with the loss of oestrogen, in particular the impact on bone, brain and heart health. Oestrogen carries a protective factor for some organs and many benefits for the body especially in women my age. Dr Louise Newson[4] reports that: *"Numerous studies have shown that when HRT is started in women who are within 10 years of menopause onset it can reduce future risk of development of osteoporosis, type 2 diabetes, osteoarthritis and all-cause mortality."*

Mentally I was as prepared as I could have been at that time. Like many opting for this invasive procedure, the reasons leading to it were far worse than the expected outcome. I was excited to be moving on and as such, eagerly anticipated surgery.

What I wasn't so prepared for was the physical slowdown I would experience afterwards, and to be honest I hadn't really acknowledged quite how major the surgery was. As someone who is not necessarily 'sporty' but is usually energetic, I expected to be back on my feet as normal relatively soon. This is what I tried to do, but on reflection, it was too much too soon.

To briefly reflect on things that would have been helpful for me to have known before the surgery, a few key suggestions immediately come to mind:

❖ That I would need to be more patient and realistic about recovery time and that I might need longer than the anticipated few weeks off from physically attending work.
❖ That I needed to be open minded on how the surgery would be performed. My operation uncovered the fact I had adenomyosis, and as my womb was enlarged,

removal via the pre-planned vaginal route wasn't an option. This meant I had a large horizontal incision across my lower abdomen and so a longer expected recovery time.

❖ That I would be scared to poop, really scared of 'what might fall out of what' if I strained (insert clenched teeth icon here) so have plenty of fibre in your diet! Smoothies, shakes, however you can ingest it. Maybe because I was using less energy my appetite decreased for a while, so I took Fybogel to top up my intake of fibre and to help keep me 'regular'. I did not want to be straining at the loo, and poop-time filled me with dread for a while even with a poop stool close by.

❖ That even though my partner was able to work from home, we should have stocked the freezer with healthy meals. Not that my partner can't cook or didn't want to cook, but my discharge from hospital coincided with the ending of a crucial work project for him. Having pre-prepared meals could have saved him time, energy and stress. Afterall, he needed to be well too.

I suspect for most people there will be a frustration with feeling held back from normal day to day activities after surgery. You know, getting about the chores, maybe having to let things go a little around the house and turning a blind eye to things that maybe matter to you usually. I'm relatively relaxed in this way anyway but even I found it challenging to have to think twice about things I took for granted.

This time of having to respect the limitations of my body gave pause for thought about all that it had given me to that point and brought thumping to my mind the reality of possible limitations of my body going forward. I felt real gratitude for what it had done for me to date and a determination to better value it in the future. Maybe I did a little bit of much needed growing-up during this time too.

On occasions when you might decide to take the recovery timeline into your own hands, think twice before you over do things. Thankfully I had no return visits to hospital, but I may on a couple of occasions have been sailing a little close to the wind.

Maybe it was the morphine but 3 weeks after hospital discharge, I took a trip to one of my favourite department stores for a facial and a Christmas browse. This foray resulted in abdominal twinges, pain and increased bleeding into my sanitary towel. Feeling faint and incredibly unwell I had to concede I should not be there. I was swiftly driven home to resume a horizontal position for a few days.

My attendance at a Christmas social around this same time is another event I should have missed. Okay, I was only there for 2 hours, but I was still clutching a cushion to my stomach at this point, barely able to fully stand up straight. In retrospect, it was a foolish decision.

I most definitely should not have undertaken a trip to London for a full day of meetings just under 2 months after my operation. On this occasion, I did once again escape a full collapse, but only just. I was bloody foolish and should have just politely declined the invitation. Travelling by tube felt gruesome. Carrying my bag and laptop around stations with stairs and not lifts or escalators was foolish.

On my return journey it was only the attentive and supportive companionship of a caring fellow passenger that kept my spirits up and stopped me from sobbing into my British Rail tea all the way back to Bridgend. It also cost me financially. I was so desperate to get home that I gave up my protest to a guard about feeling unwell much sooner than I usually would, and willingly paid the on-the-spot charge of an extra £119 to board a slightly earlier train.

Thankfully in the post-COVID-19 world, virtual meetings will hopefully be here to stay and if meetings and socials are places you need to be, then you will be able to pop into an online party in full loungewear, Thrombo-Embolus Deterrent (TED) stockings and contribute from the comfort of your sofa! We do all think we know best at times, but still, advice to not over-do things, is to be ignored at your peril. Rest assured you will know when you have done too much, as your body is good at giving you signs to slow down. The trick is not to ignore them – tetchiness, tiredness and twinges.

On the other hand, if you do experience those helpful people that like to remind you that they were back on their feet within a fortnight of surgery carrying 12kg of potatoes around whilst emptying the washing machine right after they had finished mowing the lawn (you know the type) then feel free to ignore them. Also, despite what people might comment, a total abdominal hysterectomy is **not** equivalent surgery to a caesarean-section. In one you have organs removed!

There were many items that were super helpful to have during my recovery. Bear in mind though, I had abdominal surgery not vaginal or laparoscopic, and they are different recovery processes. We also all have different backgrounds and circumstances that will invariably affect our recovery and our different thresholds of patience and pain:

❖ An over-bed trolley table. This was amazingly helpful. A hospital style table, on wheels, high enough to use in bed, super useful on those days where I didn't want to be troubling my partner constantly or frequently getting in and out of bed. In those first few weeks I had to perform some kind of commando roll to get out of bed so having useful items close by was helpful. As I returned to getting bits of work done then it was super helpful as a place to store my laptop or work on my laptop without pressure against my stomach.

- The stalwart of all post-surgery toolkits, the V-pillow. Oh, my goodness how did I ever live without one!
- Hysterectomy pants / post-operative pants – these were amazingly soft and supportive and pretty much all I wore for about 12 months. Readily available online, not cheap per pair, but worth it.
- A maternity tummy band. Both a jersey one plus a knitted one that was tighter and gave more support. These just gave that added support for my swelly-belly as I became more mobile. I did feel nervous about supporting my stomach and stitches and there was a lot of hunching and stomach clutching going on. The tummy bands really helped my confidence to just let go of holding my tum a little.
- Maternity jeans and leggings, both have soft waistbands and are easily take off and put on-able. There's a focus on comfortable waist bands and rightly so for me. Even some months after surgery, I found it difficult to endure the pressure of a jeans waistband or anything with buttons without my belly swelling up. My 'swelly-belly' was also a sign that I had done too much and often the first indication that I needed to slow down and put my feet up. I bought mine for a couple of pounds, brand new, but from a well-known clothing auction site.
- Have an extra pair of TED stockings if you can. Avoid fabric conditioner when washing them as they may lose their elasticity and compression function.
- A cushion in the car to protect under the seatbelt, especially for the journey home from hospital.
- TV subscription upgrades. I had anticipated spending my convalescence whizzing though my library of unread novels, however my focus and concentration did not facilitate this.

In amongst your pre-surgery prep, you could find out about local women's health clinics and groups. Thankfully with so many of them online now this should be an easy task, all you have to do is get the courage to join the online call. If you feel nervous about this why not take a friend to a group whether in real life or online with you for your first time, they can always leave the call once they see you are settled.

I would better prepare family, friends and colleagues about the exact nature of the surgery I underwent. I'm aware that some are still under the impression the operation I had was minimally invasive. In preparing and sharing with them that it wasn't quite that simple, I would include a copy of the recovery timeline for reference. If people know you're not fit enough to take a bath they may not expect your presence on a night out.

Be prepared for little or no follow-up support from the NHS. However amazing the service is and the workers are as individuals, I am still shocked that I was discharged without any follow up appointments in place after having major surgery. I had to take matters into my own hands, develop my own individual recovery plan and make appointments. Medically, I was given no post-surgical support other than just leaflets to take home. Below is a list of the support I pro-actively sought out:

- Consultant: I rang, advised I'd had the surgery and to request a review for HRT top-up (which needed to be carefully managed bearing in mind my hormone sensitivity) which I was granted at 6-months post-surgery.
- At my 9-month appointment I requested testosterone therapy which I was then granted at my 12-month appointment when my symptoms had not improved around cognition, energy, libido, plus I had started to experience knockout migraines.
- I started testosterone and relatively quickly recognised what I affectionately termed 'a tingle in my mingle!' ☺. It can take several months though to feel the full effect of any improvements from this therapy.
- GP: I made my own appointment with the nurse at 3 weeks post-surgery.
- Physiotherapy: a women's health physio group was scheduled from the hospital. This would have been £40 a session but the group didn't start.
- Talking therapy: a month after surgery I booked myself a couple of private counselling sessions at £40 per hour but you can self-refer in many places for talking therapies so ask at your GP practice for this information. I knew that I would likely experience a rollercoaster of emotions for a while as I moved away from the chaos of peri-menopause & PMDD and on to the new Me. I knew too that the negative self-talk I was stuck in might need challenge and coaxing to change. I'm still working on this.
- Menopause Café[5] well, just amazing! Hosting Menopause Café Cardiff has been a vital part of my toolkit in helping me not only to rebuild my confidence as I navigated through my PMDD treatment plan, but to meet so many amazing people. This is an appropriate moment to thank a few stalwarts of the Cardiff Café including Maria, Jane, Anne, Tracey, Helen W and Kathryn and not forgetting Helen from Menopause Café HQ and more recently Barbara. Thank you all for howling laughter as well as tears. You can find more about Menopause Café events online.

In doing things differently I would remove the unrealistic expectations I had placed on myself. I felt pressure to be 'better', to have recovered, to have no more emotional outbursts, to be a better mum, partner, friend and colleague etc. I didn't really allow myself to take time out for me to heal from PMDD, and I didn't put myself first nor learn to say 'no' to dashing here, there and everywhere.

What I didn't also realise then, is that my capacity to work would be much reduced for a long while, yet I was still committed to a full diary and whizzing up and down the M4 most days. I ended up just making myself more and more stressed and unwell until burnout arrived in early 2020 and I had no choice but to take time out.

Be mindful, it's easy to berate yourself for any snappy moments after surgery, but be realistic, think about the operation you have had, think about the recovery your body is going through. It's important to acknowledge the impact of the drop in oestrogen on your brain and body. For some, you may need to work through emotional traumas you may have endured in the time leading to your operation, so be kind to yourself and cut yourself come slack.

A word about this being a journey to a new you. I have found the 2 years post-surgery to be a reflective time of meaning making and self-discovery. Despite having a firm eye on my future I've had a need to try and make sense of my experiences to date. For potentially the first time in my adult life, I would be experiencing my life through a lens untainted by responses to fluctuating hormones.

What would a balanced me be like? Would I even recognise myself? Would I like myself? Would anyone else like me? This feeling of a before and an after hysterectomy life threw me off balance for a while, it threw my perception of significant events into question. My advice if you have life events and experiences you suspect might arise, then you owe it to yourself to take time to heal, and you deserve to heal.

From the confines of my bed in those first day's home after surgery, my partner seemed to be going for a home-carer-of-the-year award as he dashed up and down the stairs with cups of tea and healthy snacks, medications and injections. However, on my first trip downstairs I was witness to what was really going on. He was not actually a superhero in disguise but just someone trying to do his best for me but with too much else to do too. Right away I booked a cleaner and took the pressure off him. He was more relaxed and once a week the house was sparkling ☺.

On discharge from the hospital, I had no follow up appointment, with anyone. I felt like I'd been chopped up and tossed out with all my insides wobbling about. I made an appointment with my practice nurse just to check the wound and have a general health check. This showed I was recovering exceptionally well, no doubt largely a result of the excellent care from my partner. In attending any follow up appointments it's good to have a pre-appointment checklist. A GP has only a short amount of time to assess everything about your needs, so the more prepared you are the better.

Here are some of my tips when seeking medical guidance about your symptoms:

- ❖ Prepare well, knowledge is power. Ask your practice who is the best GP to see about menopause, do they have a menopause specialist in the practice?
- ❖ Ask your practice about extended appointments if you need more time.
- ❖ Use a symptom tracker App, print off your results to share. Have a think about environmental changes that may be going on for you too if your symptoms have changed, particularly relating to stress and anxiety. What has changed for you at home? Are you supporting anyone else right now? Are your relationships doing okay? Are you giving more support out than you're receiving? Is work okay? Money?
- ❖ Make a note of what you have already tried in attempt to manage your symptoms, e.g., medicines, herbal supplements, exercise, mindfulness activities, talking therapies etc.
- ❖ Know that it's okay to self-advocate for your health and it's okay to ask questions about your treatment plan. Until there is a mandatory menopause component in the medical education curriculum, GP's might actually know less than you do about surgical menopause!
- ❖ That it's definitely okay to question if you suspect personal opinions on HRT treatments are influencing the options you're being presented with instead of those outlined in the NICE[6] guidelines.
- ❖ If you are interested in receiving testosterone take along an appropriate report or article in support of the use of this not-yet licensed product for women. NICE guidance (NG23) on menopause states that testosterone can be considered for those that need it and can be prescribed on the NHS if the prescriber is familiar with it and is willing to prescribe it off-licence[7]. Some prefer not to take this decision and refer to a specialist for advice before prescribing. Other GPs will have prescribing restrictions which mean they are not able to offer it.
- ❖ Make a list of the questions you want to ask.
- ❖ If overwhelmed, take someone with you or have them sit with you during the call.
- ❖ Try to avoid leaving an appointment until you're feeling desperate or hopeless about your menopause symptoms. This could make it more difficult for you to take up activities that will positively benefit your wellbeing.

In moving on from my surgery, I'm looking forward to this phase of acceptance of my surgical menopause status. I'm embracing the new me and all that I need to stay healthy and well. Self-care is at the top of my list of daily considerations. I'm now taking steps that my future self will be grateful for. So, that's not a bubbly bath and a bottle of wine. It's a walk, *then* a bubbly bath, and probably a cup of tea (Oolong is my current favourite) that will help keep my digestive system ticking over whilst promoting a sense of calm.

I'm eating well, moving more, taking more notice of my body and prioritising my health over being busy. Knowing the long-term health risks relating to the top causes of death for females, I will also be continuing my HRT regime for as long as the benefits outweigh the risks. My consultant concurs there is no arbitrary reason for me to stop. Because of my sensitivity to fluctuations in my hormone levels, on discharge from the consultant's clinic, I requested a letter be sent to my GP. I wanted to ensure there would be no sudden changes made to my medication regime due to a lack of awareness about my condition or menopause treatments.

Alcohol may have to go for good. I like the new me and the decrease in brain fog from improved sleep, better nutrition and *Soberista*[8] lifestyle. I would not be giving myself the best chance to thrive if I ignored the clear improvement in how much better I can function without alcohol.

I've already mentioned Menopause Café, but other forums are available, so reach out for connections as much as you need to. If you don't already have people you regularly see in your life, this can make a huge difference in building your resilience and successfully managing your surgical menopause. If possible, find an online support group that you can join ahead of time.

A commitment to more physical activity is included in my self-care plan, and a huge positive of surgical menopause is no more bloody periods! Before surgery, as a result of adenomyosis, I was experiencing heavy bleeding for at least 2 weeks of each month. This meant every time I took up some form of physical activity it was thwarted by my periods and PMDD. Now I can just say, let's go for a walk and we can set off without me thinking twice.

This new phase of life is one without the stresses of navigating through all the crap that has gone before. I can focus more on me, I can focus on my self-development, including continuing education. We often put more thought into planning a holiday than we do into how we are going to look after our long-term health and wellbeing. After my experience with burnout in 2020, I can't stress how important it is to self-educate as much as you can on your health. It's a responsibility to yourself as well as to the people who care about you and depend on you.

Social media forums are fantastic for reducing isolation and providing opportunities to connect and make new menopause friends, but they are not spaces for obtaining qualified individual medical guidance. You can help be more prepared by reading as much as you can from reliable sources. If you are looking for good guidance about hysterectomy and surgical menopause, use recognised sites such as those of IAPMD[2], BMS[9], and WHC[7], where content is fact-checked by medical professionals.

You can also follow various medical practitioners on social media, some of whom have themselves experienced the rigours of surgical menopause and are working hard to raise awareness and share facts and helpful information. On some occasions you may even be able to chat directly with or watch a webinar featuring a qualified menopause specialist. Bear in mind though, even if you enter into an online Q&A, it's important to remember that a GP on a webinar does not have your medical history.

Reflecting on how I am today. As I write this, I am 730 days in surgical menopause. Yes, it's my 2 year "hysterversary" today, 29 Nov 2020! And no, I shall not be celebrating with a glass of bubbly. It's 102 days since I last sniffed a whiff of alcohol and right now this is the approach that suits me. Today I will finish this chapter draft for submission then head out for a walk with nothing stronger than an Oolong tea to fuel me. I may raise the excitement levels this evening though, with my knitting needles at full clack, and no I am not joking. I am enjoying living life at a slower pace and with a happier face.

Life since surgery has changed, and in every way for the better. The last two years have not been without challenge, but I have finally acknowledged and embraced the lifestyle changes I need to make in order to have the best chance at living well in this next phase.

For my partner. My partner is not a man who would appreciates a huge outpouring and PDA, however his care of me on my return home from hospital was incredible. I am a very lucky person to have had this care and I credit his attention as being part of the reason I healed physically so well and am being given space to find the new me. I just say thank you to him for allowing me time and space to heal and I do think we are closer for the whole experience. And for my children, you both inspire me to be a better person and I am just so proud of the kind, thoughtful people you are.

In closing my contribution, although I would rather avoid political statements in a helpful book, the activist in me can't say nothing! That we are having to write this book at all, driven from a need to fill gaps in lack of education and provision of accessible and relatable information and resources, is a political health inequality issue. We must have mandatory menstrual wellbeing education in schools in Wales as well as on medical curriculums to avoid many other people experiencing lost years from misdiagnoses or undiagnosed PMDD. Early intervention is key to better recovery and if this had been the case for me maybe I would not have needed this surgery. In Wales we have the #TeachMenstrualWellbeingWales hashtag, please follow, support and share.

And lastly if you are quicker, or slower to recover than someone else, who cares? As long as you feel healthy and well and can thrive not simply survive, that is what matters. You have the right to experience your recovery in your way! More importantly whilst the world is rushing you back to busyness remember you have the right to recover full-stop and keep in mind that whilst your surgery might take place over just a few hours, the impact of the quality of your recovery is long lasting. This stage can be transformational, and I wish you all the best with what comes next.

Sarah x

[1]*International Association for Premenstrual Disorders: https://iapmd.org*
[2]*National Association for Premenstrual Disorders (NAPS): https://www.pms.org.uk*
[3]*PMDD-Pod: Twitter @PmddPod*
[4]*https://www.newsonhealth.co.uk/news/making-sense-of-the-hrt-debate*
[5]*Menopause Café: www.menopausecafe.net*
[6]*National Institute for Clinical Excellence guidelines on menopause: https://www.nice.org.uk/guidance/ng23/ifp/chapter/questions-to-ask-about-menopause*
[7]*Women's Health Concern: https://www.womens-health-concern.org*
[8]*https://soberistas.com*
[9]*British Menopause Society: https://thebms.org.uk*

Sarah Williams is an Independent Equality, Diversity and Inclusion professional who provides popular EDI and menopause workshops, as well as policy development support. Following her own experiences of chemical and surgical menopause, and seeking support for PMDD, Sarah developed an interest in advocating for menopause inclusion at work and for raising awareness in the community. This has become Sarah's main focus of work. Sarah is also a seasoned facilitator of community peer support and wellbeing groups.

In early 2021, Sarah founded the Menopause Inclusion Collective, which brings together advocates, activists, menopause professionals and researchers from around the UK to advocate for, and create inclusive menopause policies, projects, resources, services and spaces.

Find Sarah at: www.equalitycounts.co.uk and www.menopausecollective.org
Sarah tweets as: @SarahLouInclude
Instagram: @SarahLouInclude

Chapter Three

Barbara Claypole, 48

Hi there, my name is Barbara, although most of my friends call me Barb, or Bee. I live in Hertfordshire with my husband Richard and we have been married for 23 years. This past year has been a lot, for both of us. Having major surgery and then a surgical menopause does not just affect you, it really does affect those closest to you as well.

My husband looked after me following the surgery and he has tried his hardest to understand the menopausal symptoms that I have experienced. However, despite the fact you may have a really supportive partner, or family, or friends to help you, there have been times during this experience that I felt completely alone, and I was not prepared for that.

Surgical menopause is sudden, and for me it hit hard and the shock of it really knocked me for six. But not to panic, as there are things you can do to help get you through it. I just wish I had known a little more about those things and what was really going to happen to my body.

It has been a little over a year since I had my total hysterectomy (uterus and cervix removed) and bilateral salpingo-oophorectomy (ovaries and fallopian tubes removed). I really want to say early on that I am so glad I had my surgery and I think it is important to get that out there before I start detailing the more challenging aspects of what surgery meant for me. It has been life changing for me in a good way. It has meant freedom from pain and heavy bleeding that were draining me of all energy and stopping me from fully enjoying life a lot of the time.

However, if I could rewind the last year and tell myself how it would be, I would say, Barb, this is going to be the hardest experience physically and mentally that you will ever have. But I would also tell myself that I would meet the most brilliant health and wellbeing professionals and make new friends who would see me through.

I described the whole experience recently as feeling as if my body was a building that had been running on full power for 47 years. Then someone pulled the plug, and the power supply was just gone. I was then left with only a backup generator to keep me going. However, I have come to adjust to that different level of power in my building and it is still open. The water supply still works, and the lights are all still on. I am not ready for demolition just yet!

I would also tell myself you will find some wonderful inspiring friends. Women who have been through this already and if you reach out that they will help lift you up when you have any wobbles or down days. I would tell myself make sure you educate yourself about the reality of surgical menopause and find out exactly what will happen to your body. Do not just rely on the clinical leaflets and booklets that are given to you. The clinical information provided in those leaflets is so important, but they really do not explain to you the detail of how it all feels, so where possible I say ask those with lived experience, not just the doctors.

First comes why? Why have the surgery?

I look back now and I knew I was at the end of the road for alternative, less invasive treatments for years and years of horrendously painful periods and heavy bleeding. Various forms of contraception including numerous pills, a coil and other medication to reduce bleeding had not worked for me. A mixture of endometriosis symptoms that plagued me in my 20's and early 30's, recurring painful cysts in my ovaries and fallopian tubes that had resulted in surgery, and with everything about my cycle and periods worsening as my peri-menopause progressed, I was ready to consider the most serious option.

I had 1 good week in a month with the other 3 weeks leaving me suffering with severe pelvic pain or heavy bleeding or both. No one knows your body better than you. I wanted it all to just stop. I remember saying to my husband, my GP and then the consultant that I simply could not do it anymore

My consultant told me that with the removal of my ovaries I would go into a surgical menopause, and if that was an issue for me and my symptoms bothered me, then we could talk about HRT after the surgery at my 6-week post-op check. At that point menopause was not really at the forefront of my mind. I was already in peri-menopause, and clearly remember thinking to myself......well, menopause is knocking on my door already, so how bad can it be to just speed things along a little? I laugh at my naïve self now looking back. I really didn't ask enough questions at the time about that element of the surgery which seems ridiculous to me now.

Those 2 words "surgical menopause" in no way prepared me for the actual experience of what was to come. I would also say to anyone about to go through this, when your consultant mentions menopause after surgery, do not do what I did and just skim over that aspect of surgery. Ask questions, research and read up about what to expect, and not just about the surgery itself.

For me at the time, it was a lot of information to take in, and understandably my consultant could not just tell me what I should do. For anyone about to make a similar decision I would recommend that, if you can, take someone you trust with you to your consultations. It really helps to have someone who knows you and what you are going through to help you decide if surgery is right for you.

Then comes the surgery and recovery!

I have found that when sharing things about my surgical menopause experience, it's important to start with and spend time talking about the actual surgery bit as so much of my overall experience began there, and even a year post-surgery I am still recovering from some of the aftereffects. I had believed the leaflets I was given by the hospital which talked about recovering in 6-8 weeks, but that is just the initial recovery from the surgery and external stitches. It takes so much more time than that to fully recover.

I think if I had been more prepared for a slower rate of recovery, it would have helped me to not feel so anxious and stressed. I just felt like a failure because I was not fully recovered and bouncing about a few months later. By knowing more about how best to handle the surgery, I could have then addressed the menopause symptoms. However, I was so concerned with recovery from the actual surgery, that initially, I ignored the signs of menopause that were hitting my body like a sledgehammer.

I remember my surgery day clearly. It started early with the usual get there and go through the paperwork admission stuff. Lots of questions and checking of blood pressure. As it wasn't my first surgery it all seemed really familiar and I was quite calm. I remember thinking only then that I am never going to have a period ever again which felt strange but also really great. The nerves really kicked in though as my husband was told to leave and I was left waiting in my hospital gown, you know the one, where your bottom is hanging out the back. I was also wearing surgical stockings which just add to the general look of 'leave your dignity at the door' when you have any surgery.

That was where I would meet the first amazing woman that helped me so much. The nurse who told me she would look after me in the coming days, Milly. I will never forget her or how she helped me and held my hand when I needed support. She was so kind but also full of joy and passion for what she was doing. There are so many Milly's out there, but she really helped me through the first few rough days after surgery.

I will never forget the stern warnings Milly gave to my husband, which was "do NOT let your wife lift a thing. Remember to be kind to her and do not let her push herself. In the coming weeks she will get to a point when she thinks she is healed and over the worst. It is your job to stop her overdoing things".

She looked at me and said, "so when you think you are ok, listen to Milly, you are not!" And my goodness she would be proven so right. You really need to be kind to yourself after this type of surgery. Rest, sleep as much as you possibly can and eat well. All of those things will help you heal faster. I have always found it so much easier to be kind to others, but not so easy when it came to myself, but this experience has forced me to change that. Self-care was and is paramount to get through everything without completely losing your mind and hurting your body even more.

If you are someone like me who has no children, as you couldn't have them, or never had them for whatever reason, be prepared that you may be given a pregnancy test before the surgery. I appreciate they sometimes do that as part of the preparation for surgery, but it took me by surprise on the actual day and I clearly recall a wave of sadness as I had a moment alone in the bathroom.

It was then that I realised my surgery was something far more than 'just' the physical removal of organs from my body. I had wanted to cry. I had accepted a long time ago that I would not be a mum, but that wave of sudden final emotion caught me off guard. But, being me, I just shrugged the feeling off and smiled as if nothing was wrong. I would have felt more prepared for that moment though if I'd known in advance that they would carry out a pregnancy test.

I personally do not do well with anaesthetics or strong painkillers. I am usually allergic to them or they make me throw up. So as expected, I spent the first day after the operation throwing up. Not exactly what you want to do after having major surgery. I was so sore and so afraid that I was going to burst my external stitches. Subsequently, I was also scared my internal stitches would also fail me and that my newly stitched up vagina would literally fall out.

I now know I am not alone in that fear as so many women I have spoken to over the last year have said that was their biggest fear too. But I wish I'd had other women beforehand to reassure me that was something lots of women worry about. Clearly though the stitches held well, but I really tested them in the first 24 hours as well as a few weeks later when I caught a cold. Sneezing and coughing left me so sore and scared for my vagina. Again! However, I reminded myself that it would be ok, nothing would fall out. I recommend if you are sick after surgery, or cough or sneeze, hold a pillow over your tummy as that helps it not hurt quite so much.

A helpful friend gave me another little practical tip before I went into hospital which I will also pass on. Make sure you take nighties with you, not pyjamas, for your hospital stay. After surgery, you might have a catheter, the drainage tube from which is harder to accommodate with PJ bottoms. Also, if you have laparoscopic surgery you will not want a waistband rubbing on your stitches and pushing on your sore and bloated abdomen.

Due to the fact that I do not tolerate strong painkillers. I relied pretty much on only ibuprofen and paracetamol for pain relief from the outset, as I just couldn't face anymore throwing up. The first couple of days immediately after surgery were tough because of that. I recall one night where I barely slept. I remember just listening to calming music and sounds of rain and the sea through my headphones and controlling my breathing, which somehow got me through.

I had learnt from previous surgeries that if you can control your breathing you really can help yourself stay calm and get through most pain when you must. I used the Calm-App[1] and it really made a difference, but I know other women have used audio books or music at that point to try and distract themselves from the initial pain of surgery.

For me, the worst thing initially after surgery was pain from the gas. They do not tell you how bad it can be, but I will. My surgery was performed laparoscopically, and they pumped my abdomen full of gas so they could poke around more easily in there, and what goes in, must come out or be absorbed by your body. The gas sometimes moves around your body, so you might get pain in your chest or shoulders and arms.

My number one survival tip is peppermint tea, which I hated, but I came to love it! It really can help to relieve the pain and promote movement of the gas. There is no polite to say this but make yourself burp and pass wind as much as you can. Just get it out. Walking helps too, moving about, even a little, as of course you won't be moving too fast in the initial days after surgery. Maybe also get someone to give you a little back rub to help try and get that gas out.

Going to the bathroom after surgery was interesting too. For me, the ability and sensation of having a wee felt somewhat different and I felt a bit numb down there at first. Something I was not aware of is that during surgery your bladder is moved about, as it can no longer rest on the organs that are removed. I now know not everyone had an issue, but I had to really concentrate to make sure I fully emptied my bladder in the days after my catheter was removed.

I have subsequently found that pelvic floor exercises are so important, and you really need to do them after surgery. Had I known beforehand how challenging that aspect of my recovery would be, I would have started doing my pelvic floor exercises a lot earlier in my life. I've also used a pelvic floor trainer since surgery. The trainer device, Elvie[2] is linked up to an App which helps gauge the strength of your muscle contractions as well as tracking your improvement over time. For me it really helped. Just keep squeezing whenever you can.

Okay. So, let's deal with this bit next while we are talking toilet stuff. Bowel movements after surgery. No easy way to say this part. It can be a little rough. Anaesthetic can make you constipated and your stomach muscles are affected from the surgery so pushing down is not a good idea. Plus, you're told that you mustn't strain <u>at all</u> due to your internal stitches. That is something that still concerns me, and you really do not get told much about that aspect of recovery when they send you home.

If you don't have a bowel movement before you're discharged from hospital, I would recommend you try and make things as easy as possible for yourself. As this was not my first laparoscopic surgery, I knew it would likely cause some issues for me and I started taking lactulose, a liquid laxative straight after surgery. That really helped. I had asked the nurses for it before I'd even had the surgery, so they gave me a laxative from day one. However, typically they don't automatically give you anything to help with a bowel movement, so I'd suggest you have a chat about it before your surgery.

In the days after surgery, I still hadn't given the menopause stuff any thought. I didn't feel any different in myself apart from being exhausted and sick from the surgery. I think it was day 3 and a cleaner in the hospital stopped at my bed for a chat. She'd had a hysterectomy a few years before and she asked me, as though we were immediate best friends because of our shared experience, "have you had your big cry yet"? I hadn't and didn't feel like having one. Not at all. I think that was the first time it hit me, and I wondered if I wasn't normal? Did everyone come out of surgery crying then, is that what surgical menopause was? I remember thinking, maybe I wasn't going to suffer at all with this menopause stuff. I even felt proud of my tough-stuff-no-crying self. How ridiculous was I? Trust me, the menopause stuff and the crying would come, just not then.

As a result of my previous experiences of laparoscopic surgery, I already knew about the stitches and the gas. When you leave hospital, you will need to invest in some big pants my friends. The Bridget Jones kind, the belly warmers. You will want to wear pants with a waistband that goes up and over your wounds and swollen belly. There will be no mini bikini briefs for a bit. So, buy some that are a couple of sizes too big for you and they will fit you perfectly while you're swollen. Comfort becomes everything. So, make sure you have some baggy outfits to wear, anything that will not put pressure on that sore tummy and the stitched areas. Also, treat yourself to one of those big triangle shaped pillows if you are having this surgery, or any surgery to be honest. They really are so comfy and they support your body.

I'd recommend you book a GP phone call appointment for a week or two after you go home from hospital, as you may need some help or advice by that point. I am so lucky that my GP is just the best; I didn't have to book an appointment as she knew when my surgery was, and she called me about a week after the operation just to see how I was. I needed that call. I'd had some issues with my external stitches bleeding, and I was struggling to sleep. I welcomed some reassurance and advice.

It's fair to say, I had not fully appreciated what having this type of surgery would involve. You hear the doctors say it's major surgery, but you don't think about what it actually means or how you will feel. But I know now, and honestly it was a little traumatic at first. I felt emotionally numb, like I was in shock for weeks after.

The physical symptoms after surgery seemed to take priority for me. I was so busy trying to get out of bed the right way, not lift anything too heavy, not pee my pants, have daily little walks or hobbles at the start, that I wasn't as aware as I perhaps should have been about the emotional and mental shifts that had started in my body. My surgical menopause was already happening, yet I wasn't really clocking the signs! I recommend you take better care of your mental wellbeing than I did at first. It's important to listen to the menopausal symptoms which can start pretty soon after surgery.

Then comes the surgical menopause!

I had already been perimenopausal before my surgery and had experienced hot flushes. My skin was a bit dry and itchy and my periods had become both shorter and longer at times and so much heavier. But that was about it.

Then I had my surgery and I literally fell off a cliff and slammed into full menopause. The clinical leaflets you get in your hospital discharge stuff are all about the surgery recovery up to 6 weeks post-surgery. What you can and cannot lift when you are recovering, and what pelvic floor exercises to do to try and stop yourself peeing your pants all the time! But that's it. No mention of surgical menopause, not one word about any of that in the paperwork.

My surgical menopause really kicked in about 3 weeks after surgery. It hit me hard, and it was a series of both physical and mental challenges that kept on coming in the months following surgery. The first actual physical symptom of my surgical menopause was something I did not even know was a menopausal thing, cold flushes! I'd only heard about hot sweats and hot flushes in relation to menopause. But I had episodes of feeling so cold. Cold to the bone. It was like someone had put me in a huge freezer without so much as a pair of gloves on. I would have to put blankets over myself just to warm up. Then, as those episodes began to lessen, the heat came. But to this day I still have both hot and cold flushes. So, get ready to literally have your body temperature go a bit haywire. Layers of clothing will become your new go-to wardrobe.

My skin became so dry, and I had a burning sensation in my mouth. My pelvic floor felt like it was on the floor, and I had a few accidents in the pee department which really bothered me. I'd never had any problems with that before and I was worried I could no longer hold onto my bowel movements either. When I needed to go to the bathroom it seemed more urgent to get there than it had ever done before.

But genuinely, the symptoms that were worse than all of those put together were the overwhelming and fast hitting emotional and mental health aspects of surgical menopause. After the hysterectomy I began to feel anxious, not about anything specific but just a general feeling of dread all the time. I was waiting all the time for something bad to happen and that was not like me at all. I really am the 'cup always half full', push-on-through in times of trouble and laugh-a-lot type of person. Where was she? Then the panic that I would never be me again hit me.

Self-doubt kicked in and I lost all confidence in myself as a person. I felt like I could not cope with anything at home or at work or anywhere else. I look back now and overall would describe it being like I'd lost all my sparkle. Even when I laughed at something funny, inside I felt no joy. I felt joyless. Not to mention the memory loss and lack of concentration, I felt like I had lost my mind. I felt more vulnerable, and not as invincible as I used to be.

I was literally desperate by the time I went to my 6-week post op check-up. I couldn't work out why I could not control my emotions in the same way I had done in the past. If I could go back to that time, I would reassure myself that it was not anything I was doing wrong or causing myself. The anxiety was not me; it was my hormones and merely my reaction to the complete and dramatic overnight loss of oestrogen in my body.

I was prescribed oestrogen-only HRT at that stage. I decided the gel form was the option I wanted to try. Patches were out for me as I'm allergic to plasters and I didn't much fancy trying to find out if HRT patches would also cause an allergic reaction. I have to say that I felt the positive effects around 3 weeks after starting HRT, and by 3 months I really felt more stable and not quite so anxious. My hot flushes reduced in number and severity and they have stayed that way ever since.

My concentration and memory have improved. However, stress and anxiety have stayed the most challenging symptoms of my menopause. I have increased my HRT dosage again in recent months and now, just over a year after surgery, I feel so much better. Better than I have felt in an awfully long time, which is amazing. But it has taken nearly a year to get my dosage right and to really feel more balanced. My advice, if you do decide to take HRT and at first it doesn't succeed, keep trying. When you get it right for you, it is a game changer.

HRT alone was not the answer for me. My number one best thing to do for my wellbeing after my hysterectomy and when surgical menopause hit, was walking.

And it still is. It is the best exercise after a hysterectomy, even when you may not feel like it. It has helped me look after and repair my body, but I also enjoy the time it gives me to think and feel what I need to feel.

Walking has given me the time and space to accept the things that have happened to my body, both physically and emotionally. I had a good few walks and cries in the early days, and I highly recommend this activity, especially while listening to your favourite music. Music helped lift my mood or helped me cry and get it all out. You really do need to have a good cry whenever you want to after your surgery. When I felt I was done crying, music then helped lift my mood. It reminded me of the happy, funny, more carefree me. She was still in there, just a slightly amended version maybe.

Complimentary therapies were not really something that I had invested much time in when I was working full-on in senior roles, commuting and living what I now describe as my old more manic life. In more recent times though, I have found something that has helped make me feel calmer and feel stronger, Reiki.

Reiki therapy has enabled me to listen to my body, and during a session I seem to know what areas of my body are in trouble or need some attention. My Reiki therapist has really helped me with this, and her empathy and kindness were exactly what I needed. I did not realise how much I needed it.

So, I would say be kind to yourself, find a way to listen to your body and to what it needs during this time. Or if like me you find that hard to do, find someone that can help you get better at it. I have learnt that ignoring symptoms and feelings will not make them go away. You need to manage your menopause, or it can be overwhelming.

A word of caution - watch your posture. After surgery you may not even realise but you will hold yourself differently as you try and protect your abdomen while it heals. I did not realise at the time, but I stayed slightly hunched forward when I sat down for months after my surgery and had spent way too much time in front of my computer. A year after my hysterectomy, I had to seek treatment from an osteopath who told me how many women suffer trapped nerves in their neck and/or back after this type of surgery due to that change in posture.

At times I felt I was going to have to say goodbye to my former self, and in a way, I have. Your body is not the same and you will not be the same after surgery. But for me perhaps that wasn't altogether a bad thing. Although I did have a mourning period for the old me.

And now, it's over a year since surgery and I'm managing my menopause by taking HRT, adding some supplements (magnesium, vitamin D, cod liver oil) and listening to my body. I am now in a much better and healthier place than I have been for a long time.

Talking has been the biggest healer for me though. On the days I felt like I could not get through this myself, having support from others who understand and can truly emphasise has been the single most important tool in my menopause toolkit. I found the online community Menopause Café as my safe space to meet other women who knew how I felt before I even said it. Speaking to a peer group about symptoms and feelings in a non-judgemental way is so liberating and I have also found some true friends from this who have helped me re-build my confidence and by doing so I have discovered a new passion to spread knowledge, information and support to other women.

Over the last 15 years I had commuted to London every day, working in senior management roles leading amazing teams of people. But in the last year that part of my life has also changed beyond recognition. The physical and mental challenges since my surgery made me question whether the sort of professional life I had was now making me happy, or more importantly, healthy.

I am currently in the process of seeing if, moving forward, this has all helped me to discover a new career. Becoming a menopause awareness advocate has been such a positive experience for me and since I left my job, due to redundancy during the COVID-19 pandemic, it has given me a unique opportunity to stop, take time to consider what my working life needs to be in the future. After everything my body has been through, and recovered from, my wellbeing must now be my number one priority if I want to keep managing my menopause and live well through it.

The final things I would say to anyone who is experiencing, or is going to experience surgical menopause, is that it is tough, but I know now that it is possible to manage it and that you can change and flourish and find a new feeling of freedom.

Please be kind and compassionate to yourself as you go through this. You do not have to feel alone. You will get through it with a little help from the menopause friends you find along the way.

[1]*www.calm.com*
[2]*www.elvie.com*

Barb tweets as: @BeeClaypole

Chapter Four

Sue Morón, 57

Surgical menopause and cancer -

I am in surgical menopause because in January 2017 I was told I had womb cancer. The menopause was not mentioned, the focus was on the cancer, nothing was said or advised about the menopause other than "you won't be able to have HRT". I was aware womb cancer might be triggered by excess oestrogen and, apparently, I was past the average menopausal age, plus I'd been repeatedly told that any bleeding over 50 was cause for possible concern and that was why they were keeping an eye on me... who knew? We had a 'funny' conversation about the heaviness of my bleeding: the gynaecologist asked: "is it heavy?" I said: "what do you mean by heavy?" After all, period flow is not something that tends to come up in everyday interactions or even those with your close friends. He said "bleeding through tampons and pads" ... it was, with lots of clotting.

Prior to this, at the time devastating news, there'd been lots of mention of peri-menopause. Every time I turned up to the GP to ask could I have some help for the overwhelming anxiety and despair I felt, the tearfulness and the fatigue that troubled me and made life intolerable, I was told "it's peri-menopause", AND? "We could try antidepressants...", no thanks, I don't want to be medicated, I want to know why I feel so crap. Well "you shouldn't sweat the small stuff" i.e. get so stressed about things, she even directed me to the book of that name, WTF?! I remember walking to the local park after one appointment and just sitting there sobbing, not knowing what to do next.

At least when these feelings came back during cancer treatment, I knew I had a reason to be reeling and feeling down. Though it was difficult to disaggregate the menopause from the impact of the cancer diagnosis and treatment, the shock and the fear had a definable origin and could be explained. I had just turned 53 when I was offered an ultrasound and advised to have an exploratory hysteroscopy. The same gynaecologist, male, the majority of gynaecological surgeons seem to be male, was sensitive to the fact that I found smears really uncomfortable and so scheduled me for an investigative D&C (a surgical procedure to scrape away part of the inner lining of the womb, carried out under anaesthetic) to find out why I was experiencing heavy bleeding.

It turned out that a polyp they removed was malignant. Thankfully, this type of cancer is slow growing, but even so clinical guidelines indicate speedy treatment which I was told would be within month. You're sitting there reeling from the news that you have a killer disease, as they hand you a Macmillan booklet and run through the initial treatment you will undergo. It wasn't just a standard hysterectomy, it had to be radical: womb, ovaries and fallopian tubes and cervix because of the location of the cancer, minutely tipping into the cervix.

I was not prepared for the rollercoaster of emotions, exacerbated by the cancer trauma. I would have liked help with anxiety before I even got the cancer. I would have liked counselling to help manage the peri-menopause. I would have liked to know that antidepressants might help, it wasn't just about medicating me, how vitamins and supplements and certain foodstuffs might help. These were all things I had to find out for myself.

Things to be aware of -

No two women's experiences are exactly the same, but there are many commonalities. We can learn things from others' experiences and then try them out for ourselves, feeling less alone in trying to make sense of where we are. I was reminded of this as I sat listening to Sam Baker reading from her new book "The Shift: How I lost and found myself after 40 – and you can too". She described her feelings on finding out that she was shedding her last egg and although I hadn't thought about it in the same way, the feelings were oh so familiar.

Even though I too had never been broody, and in fact had never wanted children, I found the loss of my womb emotionally debilitating. What made it harder was the insensitivity of the gynaecological service that thought it was fine to put those of us heading for a hysterectomy in the same clinic and space as those looking forward to giving birth. I was shocked for myself, but I was haunted by the fear and pain on the faces of older women who attended the morning clinics with me, especially those bewildered souls who came alone without the handholding of a partner or friend. There we were among the bustling, fecund, happiness of swollen bellied young women.

You have to prepare yourself for insensitivities, be your own advocate and keep questioning. We don't tend to want to make a fuss. But when I was told that I couldn't be seen for pre-op screening, by an officious clerk, as I didn't have my op date despite both I and the auxiliary who'd been sent with me explaining the clinic had sent us and here were my notes, I lost it. I said I'd just been told I'd got cancer and told to come here so I wasn't leaving until I'd been seen. I was.

Make sure you understand the treatment you are being given, take someone with you to your appointments (you'll never remember everything) and write a list of questions to ask / things to clarify when you see the medical professionals as the time passes in a flash. Read all the paperwork they hand over, no matter how badly photocopied, and ask them to repeat anything you didn't follow. It's better than going home wondering and worrying.

Remember that medical professionals have seen everything and although this can help it also means they might expect you to know something you don't. For example, they might tell you that you are sown up after surgery, at the top of the vagina. Oh yes? So "where is that reddish brown discharge coming from? Have I torn something?" "Oh that's just the stitches dissolving...."

They use gas to inflate you for surgery so they can move everything around more easily, this will lead to inevitable wind after the surgery and most of us find we are quite windy thereafter. The pelvic floor exercises you are given and should do after surgery will help remove some of that too. Drink plenty of water when you come around as it helps flush your system.

Getting out of bed can be a challenging. The knack is onto turn on your side, bend your legs and allow them to drop over the side of the bed, pushing against the bed with your arms, so you tip upright without putting strain on your damaged tissues. An auxiliary had to tell me this after watching me struggle upright.

One of the most shocking things, for me at least, is that around the time of your surgery you are told you will be able to have sex after 6 weeks.... That really wasn't on my need to know, but rather our not really thinking about it list; you should have seen my husband's face. But I appreciate some may feel differently and be aware it will feel very different for you afterwards, especially if you have been used to deep orgasms, as your womb won't be there.

One of the other indignities is having to use vaginal dilators if you have had radical surgery for cancer, to keep the vaginal space open and make post-surgery examinations easier. These aren't issued until your healing has progressed and some of the message boards mention vibrators as a possible alternative. You will more than likely need lubricant, Sylk* is a recommended brand. You may find that initially, while your body settles, you may be more prone to cystitis and yeast infections. If you feel uncomfortable, get yourself checked out.

Post-hysterectomy you may have to wait for histology results. This will be a nerve-wracking experience and, if this is the case, you should have been given the number of the nurse team who are looking after your post-surgery follow-up. Ask if not. Don't be frightened to bother them with worries or to chase results, nothing is too daft, though your GP may also be able to help, it depends on your relationship.

You may also be sent home with anti-blood clot injections (in the belly fat every night for several weeks, and yes it stings) and a spare pair of compression socks (one to wash and one to wear). Make sure you are given a sharps bucket too and know where to return it once you're done. It can feel like this stage will last for ever, but it won't. Try and enjoy some time out of your busy life.

They will tell you to rest and build up your exercise and you won't be able to drive for several months. When you do, you'll realise how much you need your core muscles for that trip out, another reason to do the gentle stretches and pelvic floor exercises you will be given.

If you already have any musculoskeletal problems, ask to see a hospital physiotherapist for advice before you are discharged which will be almost immediately after surgery, they don't hang around and tend to aim for the next day.

You will feel battered and bruised and probably as weak as a kitten. Around the third or fourth day after surgery you will feel retched as the chemicals and adrenalin leave your body. Be gentle with yourself and yes you won't be able to comfortably and safely lift a full kettle.

You will probably need help to climb in and out of a shower that is plumbed over a bath, slipping and jarring yourself is an understandable fear. Building a routine that includes getting up, showering, doing something creative and walks of slightly increasing lengths will help build your strength and benefit your mental health, as will meeting friends and a change of scenery.

You may need to get used to people telling you that you look well. They mean well, but there's always the underlying unsaid "for a cancer patient / for someone who has had surgery". But looking well and feeling well are two different things. The sudden drop in hormones may leave you as anxious and bewildered as I felt and incredibly fatigued.

I read about the extra pressure my liver was under as my body shed those hormones and so put myself on a course of milk thistle tincture morning and night and didn't drink alcohol while I was doing it, to help support my liver. I already drank lots of water so I treated myself to some fruit cordials to make life a little more interesting. My sister turned up with a great variety of non-caffeinated fruit and herbal teas as it turns out caffeine doesn't help hot flushes and certainly provoked mine. I gave up coffee for a while, and after my morning breakfast tea I found it helped to swap to the non-caffeinated variety.

I read about the benefits of sage to stave off hot flushes and ginkgo to combat the brain fog and incorporated them into my regime. I already knew about the likelihood of vitamin D deficiencies, its benefits for overall health and the use of magnesium for twitchy legs and aches and pains, but these two become even more necessary in menopause. Magnesium can help with your sleep which can be disrupted by sweats and bladder emptying and circular thoughts; many advocate taking it in the evening as a consequence. Both have been found to support your mental health, as does good gut bacteria. A probiotic post-surgery, when you have been filled full of antibiotics that can kill off the good stuff, is a worthwhile investment too.

As I wasn't able to take HRT, I had to work out how my diet might help me. Reading people like Dr Marilyn Glenville and Susun Weed told me about the power of phytoestrogens contained within flaxseed (ground to aid digestion), chickpeas and soya. Plenty of fresh fruit and vegetables, nuts and seeds that are full of minerals, wholegrains and some fish. This wasn't a problem, that was my diet anyway. The trick is to eat moderately and regularly to avoid blood sugar dips/surges that could also trigger hot flushes. I had to decide what to do about alcohol, which isn't recommended, and decided moderate would suit me better than none.

Eventually I decided to accept the offer of antidepressants to take the edge off the anxiety and help with the hot flushes. You can look up and ask for advice as to which might help you if that's a road you want to go down.

Additional support needed at work, at home -

There is no doubt that what you are going through leads you to question your sense of self, though as I have already mentioned, it was difficult to disentangle the impact of the menopause from the cancer. I struggled as do many of us. I was offered and took up counselling as part of my cancer treatment, and returned to the crafting and writing of my adolescence. These helped me decide what I needed to do next. While I'd always planned to return to working full time, not many of us can afford to leave paid work in our 50's, it was not easy, and I would have liked to have been able to afford to take more time to heal. If you can afford to take more time off or have a staggered return, do, it will benefit you in the long run.

What I hadn't counted on was the fact that things had changed and moved on while I had been absent, plus there wasn't a lot of sympathy for someone with less energy than before, so it was difficult to reintegrate. While the need for aids and adaptations is theoretically understood with respect to disability (my new status as someone having been diagnosed with cancer), the fact that you don't look any different and that the needs of women going through menopause is only just beginning to be addressed in the workplace, can make things tricky.

I got advice from the occupational health specialist at my workplace and I was glad I was in a union when I needed help. It was difficult to articulate my needs as I felt things were still changing for my body, that this was a process, I had no idea how long it would take; this did not endear me to an employer who wanted definite timescales. I did take advantage of counselling offered: it was useful to have someone out of the management loop to talk to. I wasn't lucky enough to have a menopause group in my workplace to join.

If it all gets too much, don't be afraid to ask for reduced hours, an alternative role, or move on. You will start to feel better at some point soon and quite frankly it was quite a relief to not have to be so driven. The counselling helped with the sense of failure that felt overwhelming at times and helped me see, as cliched as it might seem, this was just another phase of my life, I had nothing to prove. It made me consider what I wanted to do with the next part of my life and what was important.

At home I had to learn to ask for help, rather than just getting on with things myself and not to worry if things didn't turn out the way I usually liked them. My husband was great and there for me every step of the way, when he couldn't my sister stepped in. I had to learn how to just be, rather than always be on the go, doing things: tidying, sorting, cooking, washing and so on.

Menopausal survival kit:

Consider what you can do to support your mental health. I found the following helped:

- ❖ Books: losing myself in a great story or just finding out more about this stage of my life.
- ❖ Journaling and creative writing. I took part in online groups such as Writers HQ[1] and took the opportunity to visit book festivals and take part in online events. Take a look at Mslexia[2], For Books' Sake[3], Arvon[4], Spread the Word[5] and other regional writing development agencies.
- ❖ Walking or just being in nature.
- ❖ Swimming and stretching every morning.
- ❖ Crafting: the creation of something beautiful and colourful, for myself or someone else.
- ❖ Baking: the smells and sense of completion are wonderful; the treats are an added bonus.
- ❖ Drop into a Menopause Café[6] locally or online. You don't have to say anything, but you might hear something that helps you.

What helps on a difficult day?

A warm bath (salts relax the body), a walk in the sunshine and/or by water, a hug from my beloved and a sharing of my worries/feelings, a warm drink and a homemade biscuit, tidying up or pottering, writing out my feelings and worries, some crafting in front of a good film, lying under a blanket on the sofa watching catch-up tele, more sleep, talking to a friend, helping someone else.

If you are being advised to get a hysterectomy make sure you ask questions, ask what the options are, ask what the treatment pathways are, ask for physio advice and counselling post-surgery. The positive of my menopause experience is that I've been forced to get off the treadmill, to get back in touch with what matters to me.

Be aware that it's a rollercoaster ride, your body feels like it's fighting you all the way, you wonder how so many women have gone through this and yet it's spoken about so little. I recognised my desire to retreat to the darkened room I saw my mother retire to, but I resisted because I did not want to sink into those depths of despair, I knew how that ended. I took advice, I asked for support, I spoke to my partner, who has been wonderful.

I wondered why women at work, who had clearly reached this stage in their life, were so unable to empathise with me when I was feeling so fatigued and tearful from treatment and hormonal imbalance. I seized on the positive "it's time to reinvent yourself" messages that previously had seemed so flaky, thanking the powers that be for the resources to be able to step back and regroup. I sought like-minded souls and nurturing environments. I examined my own mortality and what makes me, me. I reconciled myself to the inevitable weight gain and shared stories and journeys. I fought the brain fog and researched what could help me weather this storm.

Here are some resources I found useful for menopause:

❖ Natural Solutions to the Menopause, 2013 Marilyn Glanville. Rodale. https://www.marilynglenville.com/
❖ Making Friends with the Menopause, 2017 Sarah Rayner with Dr Patrick Fitzgerald, 2017. Creative Pumpkin Publishing. https://www.sarah-rayner.com
❖ New Menopausal Years: Alternative Approaches for Women 30-90: The Wise Woman Way, 2002 Susun Weed, Ash Tree Publishing http://www.susunweed.com
❖ Menopause: The Change for the Better, 2018 Deborah Garlick (*Ed*) Green Tree. Also check out Henpicked online: www.henpicked.net

- Menopause clinics are few and far between so take a look at: https://www.menopausedoctor.co.uk/ & https://menopausesupport.co.uk/
- Exercise, as well as good diet, is important to help with the weight, so if you're finding it difficult this company might help: www.menohealth.com
- The Surmeno Connection, online resource and support group for women in surgical menopause www.thesurmenoconnection.com

For info about & support for those with cancer:

- Lots of clinical and lifestyle resources at https://www.macmillan.org.uk
- Cancer on Board www.canceronboard.org
- The Eve Appeal https://eveappeal.org.uk/
- www.gogirlssupport.org
- Womb Cancer Support UK www.wombcancersupportuk.weebly.com
- Action on Womb Cancer www.actиononwombcancer.org.uk

For mental health support:

- Mindfulness for Health. A practical guide to relieving pain, reducing stress and restoring wellbeing, 2013 Vidyamala Burch and Danny Penman. Piatkus https://www.breathworks-mindfulness.org.uk
- Action for happiness www.actionforhappiness.org
- The Blurt Foundation https://www.blurtitout.org/
- Midlife Meditations www.midlifemeditations.com
- For positive support through this stage of your life, take a look at: www.magnificentmidlife.com

[1]https://writershq.co.uk/
[2]https://mslexia.co.uk/
[3]https://forbookssake.net/
[4]https://www.arvon.org/
[5]https://www.spreadtheword.org.uk/
[6]www.menopausecafe.net

*www.sylk.co.uk

Sue Morón is a dual heritage (English and Spanish) cisgender woman, with friends around the world. Sue was born a northerner and has never lost those vowels, although now there's a good bit of midlands in there as well. Sue is a writer, researcher and tech savvy educational developer who has taught in secondary, adult and higher education.

Chapter Five

Charlie Barber, 46

"Well, nobody prepared me for that!" is what springs to mind when people ask me about being thrown into surgical menopause.

Could I have prepared myself better, no I do not think so. Right, let's reword that sentence. Do I think that the professionals could have prepared me better? Absolutely, and to be perfectly frank, I personally think they failed me at the time I needed professional guidance the most. So here I am, a year down the line and still battling. Battling on a day-to-day basis with my hormones, or should I say, the lack of them.

I had my surgery in 2019 at the ripe old age of 45. This was on the back of having years of numerous treatments for a raft of gynaecological issues which included: constant heavy bleeding for weeks on end, CIN3, various polyps (which were removed, sometimes without me being anesthetised), countless ovarian cysts (which ruptured), as well as eventual removal of my right ovary and fallopian tube. I'd had a cyst on my right ovary which resulted in my tummy being the size of me at approximately 6 months pregnant.

At the time my right ovary was removed, I was told this would not have an impact on me. I would confidently be able to carry on as my body would adapt even though I would only be working off one ovary for the rest of my life. However, unfortunately for me, the one ovary that was left, failed me fast and wanted to keep blessing me with additional cysts.

So, now we are up to speed on the years before my operation, it takes me to the weeks leading up to the operation itself. Now, I had the most lovely gynaecologist. When I walked into the consultation room, he read my notes, and asked how I could have been walking around like that for all those years. He said the only way to put paid to this was to have a hysterectomy, which included the removal of the cervix and remaining ovary & fallopian tube.

I was already on a low dose of HRT, because for the year or so leading up to that point, I'd experienced hot flushes, brain fog and insomnia. When I asked about the effect of surgical menopause, I was told that it would be no different to what I was experiencing already in terms of menopausal symptoms. I would have to be on HRT for the next 10 years or so as it would help to protect heart, brain and bone health. This was because I had not reached the 'desired' age of the menopause, so for protection I would 'HAVE' to have HRT. I really didn't think much more of it, especially with the forthcoming operation looming. My primary concern was dealing with the recovery itself and not what would then follow.

Operation day came, and after quite a few hours in theatre and then recovery, I was taken back to the ward. This was when it happened, this was my 'MENOPAUSE DAY!' It hit me hard and it hit me fast. The hot flushes were the worst. Do not get me wrong, I was suffering the effects of morphine and god knows what other medication I had zooming around my body, but those hot flushes were something I had never experienced before. Even the other ladies on the ward started to feel sorry for me, and then said that they hope they do not suffer in the same way. My recovery journey had now started. Sorry, when I say my recovery, I am meaning the recovery from the operation, for my journey in surgical menopause had only just begun!

The days and weeks that followed were just a living hell to be truthful. Hot flushes were frequent and debilitating, my bones and joints were hurting so much so that I would have to physically pick my legs up and swing them out of bed. My skin itched, my hair started to fall out and that's just to name but a few of the various common symptoms of menopause I found myself experiencing.

What I did not take into consideration was the feeling of being so low all of the time. The feeling of deep sadness and hopelessness. I did not realise I was falling deeper and deeper into a pit of depression which no matter what I tried to do, I could not seem to shake myself out of.

I was standing in the shower when I hit rock bottom. That moment came after days and days just sitting in the front room looking at my empty fireplace, just staring at the brick work for hours on end. I had a choice to make, I either gave into this feeling, pack my stuff and walk out on my family, job and my life which I loved more than anything, or I was going to try and get the 'Charlie fighting spirit back' and do something about the situation. I knew this was not me, this was not who I wanted to be, and that I needed to fight to get ME back!

So, this is when it started, my fight to get control of 'my menopause'. I contacted the doctor and had my HRT changed as it was clearly not working. Due to having had endometriosis (and adenomyosis, which I found out once I had my hysterectomy) I was put on a combined HRT pill to try and help prevent any flare ups.

I then read up and started my research journey, to empower myself with as much knowledge as possible, because as we know 'knowledge is power'. From this I started my own blog entitled *What Uterus?*[1] which charted my recovery step by step. The blog meant my family could know how I was doing without having to repeatedly ask me questions all the time. It also made me feel better. Firstly, by knowing I was saying how I was feeling, but also knowing it may help somebody else, like me, who was in a similar situation. I then went on the search for local support groups, which is when it came to light, that there were in fact none anywhere near me. I then knew that was what I needed to do once back on my feet.

So, this is me now, and 15 months post-op, I am now a qualified 'MenoLeader' and I run support sessions for women going through the menopause, providing fitness classes and support sessions on topics related to the menopause. I have taken various courses and qualified as a fitness instructor, given talks related to the menopause to the NHS, been a guest blogger on various women's health websites, and created various social media platforms to be able to reach as many women as possible.

Most importantly though, I have supported women in similar situations to myself. Women who like me in the beginning had nobody to lean on. I let them know it will be okay, that they are not going crazy, and that how they are feeling is in all probability mainly down to their hormones!

My menopausal journey is still very much ongoing, and I have no doubt it will have its up and downs for years to come as I still battle with my doctors over certain medications. I have tried various HRT regimes. Due to vaginal atrophy and a bladder prolapse, which was down to the hysterectomy itself and a lack of oestrogen, I now use local oestrogen as well (which is amazing). I exercise regularly as this helps my mood. Exercise also keeps a check on my weight gain and helps to maintain bone, heart and brain health.

Most of all though, my surgical menopause has given my life back to me! Seems bizarre right?! After being determined to become a headteacher for years and gaining my headteacher qualification, I realised quickly after my operation, I could not keep up anymore. The brain fog was so horrendous, I felt inadequate at my job and I felt I'd aged at least 20 years overnight since my operation. The moments of being in meetings and not remembering what I was talking about, or having words and names fall out of my brain was now happening to me on a daily basis. I'd always prided myself on having an outstanding memory, but my memory became terrible. This became all too apparent when I was driving to the doctor's surgery and had to pull over as I couldn't remember where I was driving to. I just wept on the side of the road. At one point I actually thought it was the onset of Alzheimer's. But I now know it was not, it was just my hormones!

So, as I am writing this final part of my story, I'm preparing to step down from being a deputy headteacher in the school I have been a part of for the last 18 years. I re-evaluated my life and decided I want to be back in the classroom full time. It's the place I love being the most, to educate, and where I only need to worry about the students in front of me rather than the whole school.

I decided to simultaneously push forward with my work for MenoHealth[2]. This allows me to support women going through the menopause, support more women like me, empowering them so they are given the best choices and support for their own menopausal journey. This was something that I did not have when I first embarked on my own journey. Doing all this though, meant I had to give up something, and that something was being a deputy headteacher.

My passion has now been ignited for helping others, helping to empower women, educate people about the menopause and break that taboo. Nobody should feel like I did, and nobody should feel that they need to walk out on their lives because they feel so desperate and do not know what's happening to them. This is just not for me, this is for my daughters and my daughters daughter's, this is for generations to come.

I have been asked this question many times, would I agree to have my hysterectomy if I had my time again? Absolutely yes, as it has been life changing for me, but more so for the better. Remember, menopause changes lives, but it does not have to wreck lives.

[1]*What Uterus blog: http://whatuterus.com*
[2]*MenoHealth https://www.menohealth.co.uk*

Charlie (likes to think she is 30, feels like she is 80 sometimes) Barber describes herself as "a mother, wife, daughter, sister, friend, deputy headteacher, MenoLeader, blogger and crazy menopausal woman".

Website: www.cvbbalancedhealth.co.uk
Find Charlie on Twitter: @UterusWhat and @MenoLeaderCB and @CvbHealth

Chapter Six

Hayley Burridge, 42

"It's ok to rest as nothing in nature blooms all year round"

I am married with two children and was diagnosed with premenstrual dysphoric disorder (PMDD) in 2018. In November 2019, I felt hopeless, I felt useless and every day I felt the precious life I'd been given was unbearable. I had everything yet I felt nothing. I had been surviving behind a thick sheet of glass with my feet cemented in a slow-moving wave of sand and treacle, unable to reach out to anyone or hang on to anything.

That was the life I thought I deserved, was given, had to survive through. As long as everyone else was okay, as long as they liked me and were happy with me, taking from me, draining me, then that's what I was there for. And I wasn't in control of any of it.

After long and exhausting years of people-pleasing, masking my feelings with no self-care or regard for myself, I began to completely lose myself and my purpose. I'd learnt my dearest mother had cancer, watched her suffer, watched her die and I'd not allowed myself to grieve in my unique and natural way. Instead, I behaved in the way I felt I was expected to. Rightly, wrongly, unintentionally that's what I let happen, as then, I didn't know any other way.

I was, and still am, naturally caring and genuinely friendly and always put the feelings and expectations of others before my own wellbeing. Unbeknownst to me at the time, I was living with the beast that is PMDD. It heightened my depression and anxiety and led to two breakdowns and many episodes of feeling suicidal. Even though I had everything, I felt nothing.

I had been morphing into someone else for a long time. For reasons that I can only guess at, people just didn't know what to do with me and that still hurts. There is so much stigma surrounding mental health and hormonal health. I feel I was left with an element of post-traumatic stress due to the lack of knowledge and communication within the healthcare system about PMDD, surgical menopause and the lack of aftercare.

The best way to explain my life with PMDD before surgery, was that every 2-3 weeks, I would hit a self-destruct button. I literally let my life, my normally very happy and satisfying life implode around me. Then, when the dark thoughts lifted and cleared completely, I'd spend the next few weeks trying to pick up the pieces before I went through it all again. Exhausting

My emotional experiences with PMDD included: extreme mood swings, feeling upset, angry, irritable, hopeless, overwhelmed, extreme anxiety and depression, difficulty concentrating, no or little energy, no interest in life, extreme fatigue, and suicidal ideation. Amongst my physical and behavioural experiences were: severe headaches, breast tenderness, feeling bloated, overeating, and being very difficult to work or interact with. I now believe that my PMDD was the culmination of three things:

I.   genetic predisposition e.g., sensitivity, inflammation etc.
II.   physiological & hormonal trauma e.g., difficult childbirths
III. psychological trauma e.g., relationship difficulties, bereavements

After numerous appointments and exhausting conversations with GP's and trying out different types of antidepressant, I eventually broke down and desperately tried to explain "I know my body, this is hormonal and cyclical". I was immediately given an urgent appointment at the nearest mental health unit as the doctor felt I was a risk to myself. At that stage I was desperate. I was interviewed. The conclusion was I just needed a different medication and I needed to attend a course on 'activating my life and wellbeing' run by the local council.

I attended the course and gave 100% even though I struggled through the days when I was very symptomatic. My advice to the 'struggling me' would be to provide the GP with a detailed record of symptoms for several months. PMDD is still not very well known amongst health professionals and getting a diagnosis for PMDD can be a very slow and frustrating process. I was diagnosed with PMDD by a psychiatrist, advised to attend a stress control course, and referred to a gynaecologist.

I was put on a drug to induce a temporary chemical menopause. Within a few days I went from managing and coping, to being plunged into a dark ravine of uncontrollable thoughts about death. It was like an out of body experience. I wanted it all to stop, I had had enough. I wanted to get off NOW. What use was I to anyone? I was just upsetting my husband and children as I couldn't function the way they needed me to. I couldn't enjoy the nicer side of life so what the hell did I have to look forward to? I ended up in A&E and then in a mental health unit. My experience there haunts me even now. At the end of it, I was simply discharged feeling the same way I had before I'd attended A&E, just more exhausted, disappointed and of course traumatised.

Why isn't there someone like a hormone/menopause/mental health care worker who can intercept women at A&E when they present with hormone related emergencies rather than letting them experience unhelpful services in the wrong department? What I would have given for a friendly faced nurse to have held my hand and reassured me that I was going to be okay. Instead, it was one consultant after another who had never heard of PMDD and who asked me the same questions over and over in that tired 'end-of-shift' manner.

At one point I had arranged to be seen at my GP's surgery for a regular injection. Up until that particular appointment, I had previously always been given the injection into my arm muscle. However, a nurse gave me the injection into my belly fat. When I asked why, the nurse explained that by injecting into my belly fat, the drug travelled around my body a lot slower, and that should help prevent the massive high and low fluctuations of hormones to which I had an extreme sensitivity (thanks to PMDD).

I bled throughout my hormone injections which lead to untreated anaemia. However, the hormone specialist had advised me on numerous occasions that I couldn't be bleeding as my ovaries had been temporarily chemically turned off. Where does one go from there?

I had been passed from pillar to post in between PMDD diagnosis, hormone injections with specialists, the GP and the gynae-consultant. That not only contributed to my anxieties, but I felt I was a trial, a statistic, an inconvenience even, and my treatment turned out to be one big trial and error. Numerous times I presented myself to the clinic in a highly emotional state. I remember thinking "I can't go on like this, there is just no empathy or understanding coming from anywhere….is it me? Am I just a joke?" If I had to give advice to a younger me, I'd say don't be afraid to ask questions. It's your body, and you know yourself best.

The support from the gynae-consultants was invariably always the same, due I felt, to a lack of communication. I would turn up for appointments armed with a file full of notes, appointment letters and such like, only to leave feeling emotionally drained, unsure of what was next and disappointed at the lack of care and support. Throughout my whole experience I never felt "looked after" and that surely isn't right or fair. I actually went back to a GP in a state of desperation only to be told, "if you're not actively suicidal there is not a lot I can do".

I went armed to one appointment with all my information, just praying I was going to get some sort of help with how I was feeling. The doctor explained coldly, that due to the pandemic and waiting lists, cancer patients were being prioritised, but she was happy to refer me privately. I left in tears, angry and felt guilty that I thought my hysterectomy was more important than a cancer patient.

I am now recovering from a hysterectomy which took place on 19th October 2020 when I entered into a strange new world of surgical menopause. Before my hysterectomy, I'd left my job of 17 years and I was painfully learning about so many triggers that were making me feel unwell on a daily basis. In my experience, education and communication are paramount and within my world at the time there was very little of either. That resulted in me withdrawing further into myself. I'd questioned my relationships and why I'd always felt like "that elephant in the room". Years of suffering, undiagnosed and desperate.

I was 42 at time of my surgery and I tried my very best to prepare myself both physically and mentally by keeping my fitness levels up, eating well, meditating, journaling, practicing self-care and building up my knowledge by reading positive stories of other women who had gone through the same procedure.

I was eventually lucky enough to have my hysterectomy performed laparoscopically, and at 3 weeks post-op I felt really well, everything was healing nicely. Having had a caesarean section previously, I was very happy not to have had a more invasive surgical procedure. There was an issue with poor communication around my HRT dosage going forward, which was not great aftercare following such a major operation.

At 4 weeks post-op I had hot, hot flushes and night sweats. I'd started to wake feeling quite anxious again, mainly about my aftercare and HRT. Perhaps I had jumped the gun as I'd healed so well after the keyhole surgery. I had started to focus more on what the future might hold rather than taking things one day at a time. That is where self-care and mindfulness are so important. I did have an episode recently where I cried uncontrollably and that negatively impacted my family. Communication is key. Even though I'd healed well, I still needed to explain about the emotional side of surgery and menopause which isn't easy when you're feeling the way you do. I would advise having such conversations before surgery!

I believe much of my anxiety could have been avoided by having a clear understanding and plan of what to expect after surgery. The consultant spoke to me about how difficult the surgery was due to scar tissue from previous operations (caesarean section). Why couldn't he have taken the time to say *"okay so going forward you will be in my care with regards to recovery and an HRT plan. I will be in touch to arrange a follow up appointment where we can discuss your surgical menopause, what to expect, how to manage symptoms and looking forward to the future"*. Okay, perhaps that's a bit too much to expect but something along those lines would have really helped.

At 7 weeks post-op, I woke for the first time in ages without a heavy heart and I noticed my head was no longer full of dread. Amazing! My menopause symptoms are still there but they are manageable, and I am gradually finding my way back to feeling more emotionally balanced.

Having a hysterectomy and going into surgical menopause has been life changing. For me it is a reminder that I need to regularly listen to my body and constantly make changes to ensure I stay healthy and strong throughout my post-menopausal years.

I have a very supportive partner and children. I am very lucky. I had never really stopped to think about various difficult life experiences from my past, and whilst I can't do anything about the past, I have learnt that self-care is really important for me as I move forward. My self-care includes:

- a balanced diet
- good quality 'me' time
- cut off as much as possible from negative influences
- keep on top of medication
- therapy
- finding purpose & creating a lifestyle which suits me
- positive affirmations
- quality sleep

"Be proud of who you are and not ashamed of how someone else sees you. The past was. Tomorrow maybe. Only today is".

Find Hayley on Instagram: @hayley_pmddawareness

Chapter Seven

Sarah Garlick, 44

"Let everything happen to you
Beauty and terror
Just keep going
No feeling is final"

- Rainer Maria Rilke -

There is nothing really unusual about me, I'm just your regular Sarah. To help write this chapter, we were sent various useful prompts. The first one being *'Why are you in surgical menopause?'* This is one of the most difficult and upsetting questions I ask myself, usually in the middle of an insomnia wracked night, or when I am trying to find fresh skin space on my thighs for HRT patches.

I'm trying to follow the breadcrumbs to lead me back to the beginning of this surgical menopause journey. Me and periods never got on. From day one (aged 11) we were not friends. I remember feeling bewildered that other girls could just get on with things when Aunty Flo came to visit. I remember puzzling as to how other girls could wear PE knickers without a second thought. I recall wearing multiple 'brick type' pads and living with an almost constant fear of flooding. I thought I was on my own in this personal hell. My adult self knows I wasn't. Periods left me ashen, bedridden, migrainous and mentally devastated. Every month.

At 15 I was put on the pill by our family doctor, this was to fix things. It kind of did. It wasn't ideal. I wasn't a fan. But this carried on until an upgrade to the Mirena coil after childbirth. Incidentally, throughout pregnancy, period free and with a baby in my tum, I felt fabulous.

A decision taken fairly lightly to remove this Mirena coil seems to be a significant breadcrumb. I was getting married, and at 36 was feeling insecure and desperate to shed the pounds I had piled on before my big day arrived. I do not care what doctors say, when I had the Mirena coil I only had to look at a cheese sandwich to go up a couple of dress sizes. Everything was fine, until those old teenage symptoms came flooding back. I went to the GP, I was referred to a gynaecologist who recommended an endometrial ablation. This was to fix things. The endometrial ablation was a shock to the system in more ways than one.

Yet there are more breadcrumbs. There followed a devastating increase in pain, as if my body was simply refusing to accept that periods would not be happening. I started having a new and bewildering symptom, bloating.

Next stop, a hysterectomy. This is when I learnt that a hysterectomy was 'just' the removal of my troublesome womb. The consultant confidently informed me that adenomyosis had in fact been the cause of my swelling and bloating all along. At last. A reason. This operation truly taught me the meaning of difficult recovery. I remember, on returning home, after a brutal, brutal hospital stay, shakily climbing the stairs like an octogenarian woman. The pain was unforgiving. But determined, I walked and slept and took muchos pain relief, and repeated this until I was *kind of* back to my old self. This will fix things. Except. It didn't. The pain and the bloating returned.

This time, in a new and exciting twist, I was referred to the gastroenterology department. I mean. Hey. I'll try anything. Really. This was after too many distressing GP appointments battling to be heard. One stand-out moment being when I was accused of "drinking too much fizzy pop'. As if all along, I had hidden a secret soda habit which had inflated me to Violet Beauregard proportions.

I was put through myriad of gruesome tests. There was some talk, after a session of 'biofeedback' that my pelvic floor was *too tight*. After an eyebrow raising, tear jerking endoscopy and colonoscopy, I also had a functional gut test, in which I got to drink my own bodyweight in barium and wear arse-less chaps like a nightmarish NHS version of Christina Aguilera. Never mind. This will fix things.

I was given a vague diagnosis by a disinterested gastroenterologist. The diagnosis was irritable bowel syndrome (IBS). I was given medication. I changed my diet and delved into the dastardly difficult world of FODMAPS. This will fix things.

You're way ahead of me. It didn't. If you are still reading this. Thank you. I wish I could glamorise it more. That's the thing. It was boring, I was boring. Days spent in bed are dull. You become dull. The world starts to seem dull. It gets easier to close the curtains. What I will say is one thing this whole debacle has gifted me, and what a gift it is, is finding out who your true friends are. I mean this in a positive sense, some people in my life have revealed themselves to be the kindest, most resilient kind of friends. The ones that don't forget you. Those out of the blue ones that message you. True gifts.

Onwards. Back to my weary gynaecologist, who was now barely able to hide his disappointment upon seeing me on his appointment list. We were going to get nuclear. Zoladex implants were suggested and administered. Chemical menopause ensued. This would show that things could be fixed.

I was NOT prepared. The plan was to 'turn off' my ovaries, to see if that might help with the awful bloat. And, just for laughs, we were going to do this without HRT. It only took a couple of weeks for me to lose my mind. I knew something was wrong when I started to think of jumping out of my bedroom window. I was confused, and very, very frightened. I managed to still have a little bit of me left to speak to the GP through wracking sobs. I was tranquilised. I hid away. The bloating stopped. This had (kind of) fixed things. Although, I was in possession of a relentless, racing, distressed and confused mind. The 'hot flushes' I experienced actually hurt. Nobody tells you how bad hot flushes can be, how these 'demon waves' have become a source of dismissive humour amazes me.

Disappointingly the response I got from a fair few women was a rather dark 'welcome to my world' passive aggressiveness. No matter how much I tried to explain that chemical menopause is quite different to the more normal, natural 'run up'. The fact that it can be very bad indeed if (all of a sudden) ovaries do not produce what ovaries are designed to produce. I have found the same with surgical menopause. For the first year after my operation, I felt like 'The Surgical Menopause Lady' trying over and over and over again to tell people that surgical menopause was different to natural menopause.

This has become so important to me. It is so important to me. I don't know why. I want to shout it from the mountain tops "SURGICAL MENOPAUSE IS DIFFERENT FROM NATURAL MENOPAUSE!". It's like I'm stuck on repeat. I don't know how I will ever be heard enough. Perhaps doing something like writing a chapter for a book will help.

Back to the story. It was Christmas, and I recall saying to my mum that the Zoladex implant was due to wear off on Christmas day, and as such the day could double up as a joyous end to chemical menopause. And right on cue...on Christmas night the bloating returned. By boxing day, I was in unbearable pain, desperately seeking comfort in a hot bath like a birthing hippo. This was worse than ever. I returned to the consultant. We must fix things.

The gynae-consultant was not impressed with me. In the darkest of turns, he asked whether I should go back to the gastro-department instead? Although I had spent countless hours trying to educate myself to the best of my non-medical ability, choosing where to be referred was not ideal.

Fast forward to Spring 2019, I made it up the M5 to Birmingham (via a strange, hope-destroying, eye wateringly expensive stop off to Harley Street on the way for good measure). The consultant in Birmingham oozed warmth. He was running late for our appointment, I understood why when I sat in his office. I spoke, he listened, no rush, no judgement. It was a revelation. Based on the Zoladex trial, the plan was to remove my ovaries, my cervix, any endometriosis and remaining adenomyosis. All roads had been leading to this. The final fix.

Surgical menopause was not mentioned much. Which seems extraordinary to me knowing what I know now. It was very matter of fact. At 43, with no more children to bear, my ovaries would be whipped out. I would have a 'cuff' instead of a cervix. I would be free of that mysterious cycle that had blighted my life since I was 11. The women in various communities I had joined hinted that saying goodbye to your ovaries was bad. I recall being terrified of waking up in that horrendous mental state all too familiar from my temporary chemical menopause, waking up forever changed.

Before the surgery I read, and read, books about menopause, about endometriosis and adenomyosis, and then I stopped reading. I danced between wanting to know everything and wanting to know nothing at all.

That's not to say I didn't prepare as much as I could. I had picked up a few tips along the way. In no particular order; listening to pre-surgery hypnotherapy on YouTube, an eye mask, mints, a heat pad, Gas X and Wind-Eze, smock dress (to avoid wounds), lip balm. Photos of flowers and cards sent, saved on my phone. Then all kinds of anti-constipation aids including grapes, coffee, and liquorice. A 'stool-stool', playlists, book lists, box set recommendations. Freezer cooking. Also, body spray for the hospital hum. The comfiest of pants. Moist toilet tissue. A maternity pillow. Roll on essential oils. Painkillers a-plenty. Slip on slippers and shoes.

The day before, 'Oophorectomy Eve', was bowel prep. Sounds okay. Not too bad. How bad can it be? Two drinks. That's all. That is all. As days go, bowel prep day will stay with me for life. There are no words. The only advice I can give is to stay as close to a toilet as is humanly possible. To have a toilet to yourself if at all possible. Vaseline is your friend.

I can only recall fragments of the actual surgery day. I was eerily calm. Too calm. I look back at the photos of the morning, I look at my face, and I know I am different. I have grieved, I have felt grief. I remember walking down to the theatre, offering my hand to the anaesthetist, I remember letting go. I remember coming round, I remember struggling to stay awake, I remember eating delicious apple crumble and pressing on my morphine pump throughout the night. I remember my nurse being an angel.

I remember the consultant visiting to say all went well. He let me know that if the terrible bloating came back, then there would be nothing further that could be done. He quickly scribbled a prescription for HRT, at a level that 'suits most women'.

Then he left. My sister, ever useful went to the hospital pharmacy to get the HRT, to discover that the hospital pharmacy didn't stock it. Although, given it was an oophorectomy epicentre I found this strange, and so began my battle with getting the correct HRT; another book, possibly in two volumes.

I remember the journey away from hospital, clutching a pillow and feeling every bump in the road, feeling shell shocked...wondering if/when the madness would commence. So began another recovery. I walked, I rested, I walked, I rested.

Memorably, my first GP appointment to sort out my HRT resulted in said (female) GP telling me I had not had a hysterectomy. In my 'fit your life story into a 10-minute appointment with yet another GP' skit, I had used the term 'hysterectomy', instead of bilateral salpingo oophorectomy. This was not a great time to pick at straws. The GP also accused me of demanding 'weird and wonderful things from private health care' when I asked for testosterone. That day I walked back and forth trying to get a prescription for HRT patches filled from any local chemist. That walk ruined me, in more ways than one.

For any ladies embarking on this journey, I would definitely say enquire about HRT first. That's if you can take it. I know it's not a given. It has taken me a year to get my hormone levels tested, to be prescribed a dose that makes me feel most like me, which is 250 Estradot patch twice a week. Slightly different from the '50' that 'suited most women'.

A key junction on the HRT highway was accepting that the NHS GPs could not help me. I know there are some good ones out there, but I couldn't find one. I was fortunate enough to have some finances to give me a leg up. My first step was to see Hazel Hayden, from Bristol Menopause. I could tell as soon as I saw her standing in the doorway to greet me that she was one of the good ones. Comfort radiated off her. I was heard. I was validated.

An appointment at The Newson Clinic felt like visit to a spa, for it smelt wonderful. I thought it was expensive. It worked. My memory returned. My mind has calmed. My bones no longer ached. With the right level of HRT (including testosterone I might add) I no longer felt like I was turning to dust. Yes, it had been a long year but finally, FINALLY I was fixed.

The only things different now are my ever-thinning hairline (HELP. PLEASE), chin whiskers, a suspicion of accelerated ageing (invest in a good moisturiser and bathe in it) and 'down there' is not exactly the best. Also, my inner chub is not so much inner anymore. Metabolism, where you at? But I'll take it. Fixed enough.

Things that help: exercise, exercise, exercise. Never want to do it. Always glad I did. As a counsellor who makes a living from talking about feelings, I bow down at the altar of exercise for its ability to shift mindset (and chub). I have walked, I have run, I've attended spinning classes.

The other things I have tried are; acupuncture – fabulous, if you get a good person. Chinese herbal medicine did not work for me, or my bank balance. Reflexology – now this, this is just wonderful. Yoga, a meditative practice called Yoga Nidra has given me the gift of (some) peace. If you can go to a class, great, if you cannot, try the free App 'Insight Timer'.

I have discovered The Menopause Support Network[1], HysterSisters[2] and Menopause Café[3]. I also found Bristol Menopause[4], The Newson Clinic[5], and The Surmeno Connection[6]. I have found that the state of women's health care is nothing short of a global scandal. I have found receiving messages of support from strangers who know exactly what you are going through is balm for the soul. It's the best kind of women supporting women.

Support is out there if you need it, but you must, must seek it. I have learnt to ask for help. I am learning. I have learnt that my work is an awesome place to work. They have been very understanding and enabled me to keep doing what I love. I cannot lie, I wish I had kept one ovary. Just one of the little fellas. I wish I had known.

How does surgical menopause feel? For me I feel anger bubbling away, a different kind of anger. Rage. Quiet rage. Acceptable rage? It's an anger filled with unattractive bitterness and jealousy. At 44 I did not want this. But there are those who are 34, 24... there are those who would switch their situation for mine in a precious heartbeat. I know this. I still give myself permission to feel anger, to feel bitter. Reading this back quickly, words that are coming from my fingertips, is it 'unattractive' bitterness? Where to start with that one. I feel that there is a vortex of feelings associated with menopause, it sucks you in and is self-perpetuating. I am angry and bitter about being a menopausal woman who is angry and bitter. I do not have enough energy to climb the mountain a second time for some therapeutic screaming.

I am jealous of women who aren't going through this. I am jealous of younger women, those that don't know. I didn't know. For me it connects to the ageing process, the quiet, imperceptible move from maid to maiden to crone. Although it wasn't silent nor was it indiscernible. Surgical menopause was a loud full stop after a silent snip. I am jealous of men that never need to think of this.

Then comes, sometimes, the peace, the acceptance. The snuggling down. The (more) comfortable clothes. The slightly lower heel. The slightly earlier night. Not always, but sometimes. There is a delicious warmth to be found in this. Never underestimate the comfort of this.

Every now and again when friends tell me they are having a rough time because they have their period, I feel lucky. I do not need to buy any more sanitary wear ever. Period. (Sorry, couldn't resist). My mood, my emotions, my energy are the same every day of the month. I no longer have unexpected breakdowns or fits of anger and then realise the 'when' as well as the 'what', 'who' and 'how'. I can wear white jeans. I feel completely detached, untethered to that dreadful abusive relationship with Aunty Flo. This has got to be the upside, the gift. The gift of being fixed.

On reflection, the first prompt was a great prompt. Look at all the breadcrumbs. The final prompt is a little tough *'How are you now?'* When my HRT was finally going in the right direction, I had a new lease of life. This was it. This was finally it. All those days in bed. All those days in tears. In pain. I'm going to make up for all those days, and then some. I'm going to live my life honouring the ladies I've met along the way, the ladies who I know are spending those toughest of days still in pain, trying to stay sane, searching Netflix for things not yet watched, treating themselves to fresh pyjamas, plugging in their heat-pads, looking through the window at people getting on with their lives.

2020 was going to be my year. Then came the pandemic. The irony of being locked down. Hit me up for tips I told friends and colleagues. It was ok. I had myself. I was fixed. I cracked on. Everyone is anxious. I worked. A duty shift on a warm July Friday, sat at my desk looking out at the sun.

A twinge. A stabbing pain. The disbelief. Just disbelief. Terrible Tum had returned. 'It came back today' I posted on Instagram. Numb. I was not fixed. I am not fixed. But, that is another chapter for another book, and it really does pain me to say, I don't know what that book is about.

If you are going through surgical menopause, be soft on yourself, then softer still.

[1]*www.menopausesupport.co.uk*
[2]*www.hystersisters.com*
[3]*www.menopausecafe.net*
[4]*www.bristolmenopause.com*
[5]*www.newsonhealth.co.uk*
[6]*www.thesurmenoconnection.com*

Sarah is a Senior Wellbeing Practitioner helping students to navigate this thing called life. She lives in a small town near Bristol and is married to a man nicknamed 'Gobber' on account of his goblin-ness.

Find Sarah on Instagram: @Terrible-tum

Chapter Eight

Shelley Chapman, 61

Hi, it's nice to meet you. I'm Shelley Chapman, a housewife and mum who had an emergency, total hysterectomy aged 43. I went through the menopause without HRT and came out the other side fairly uneventfully.

I had to have a hysterectomy because of the amount of pain I was in, and they couldn't get on top of it. I couldn't think straight or do much. The pain had taken over my life and something had to be done. To be honest, even though my husband was disabled (leg amputee a year and a half before) and our 3 girls were quite young (10 and twins of 8), for me, the time couldn't come soon enough. We had also just moved into a property (nearly 3 years previously) that we were renovating (just before my husband's accident) that also had a garden that looked so promising when we bought it. It had grass, lots of it for the girls to run around and a big tree that the girls could go and climb and fall out of.

Even though so much was going on, I just wanted to get my life back together, instead of being in a constant fog of pain with something I couldn't control. I nearly skipped into the hospital when they told me that it was "my time" for the op. Come the day of the operation, I realised how much I wanted it, because as the day started dragging on and the ward became more and more empty and the pain became worse and worse (I couldn't take any medication), by the time they came out and told me I couldn't have it done that day I was in tears with the pain.

That made me realise that I needed the surgery and I needed it as soon as possible. As things were, my quality of life was near zero. I was no help to myself or my family. I didn't have any female family members to talk to and possibly discuss the impact surgery might or might not have on my life. I'd sadly lost my mother within a week, one month after my 21st birthday, and unfortunately, I never saw her side of the family again. I wonder if the trauma of losing her so young, she was 49, plus the fact that my sister was younger than me, taught me to get on with things and roll with the punches.

I'd had a chat with my doctor about the hysterectomy and what my 'options' were after surgery. The suggestion was HRT. I was told I would be on it for about 8-10 years, but eventually I would have to come off it. When I asked if any menopausal symptoms would come back when I stopped taking it, I was told "most probably, yes" because HRT would be putting into my system the hormones that my body was no longer producing. I asked if it was possible to try a natural approach and if that didn't work and I was struggling, could I go back and get HRT? When the answer was "yes", that made my mind up.

My way of thinking was, if my body was trying to get used to dwindling hormones (which happens gradually with natural menopause), instead of trying to put them back, maybe there was a more natural and longer-lasting way to deal with the symptoms as and when they came along?

In many ways before the surgery, I didn't know a lot about any long-term effects that might occur as a result. And honestly, I think that was an absolute blessing. Let me explain. When you know a lot about something, you worry and wait for it to happen to you. When you don't know, you're quite blissfully unaware of what to expect, so you don't expect it and I think that's what happened to me.

Finally the day came for the hysterectomy. Whilst being wheeled down to theatre I asked for a tummy tuck at the same time. That went down like a lead balloon, so I assumed I wasn't the only one to ask. The sad thing was, I was being serious. Anyway, back to my story.

The operation was 'uneventful'. The pain was manageable. The hospital and staff were fantastic, and I enjoyed going home and being treated with kid gloves for a few days. As you can imagine though, the novelty soon wore off. Everyone got bored with doing the things they had been used to me doing and slowly life got back to 'normal'.

Because I wasn't expecting anything, I didn't know what to expect, if that makes sense. That, I think, was my saving. As the weeks and months went by, I got stronger and life went back to normal, even without the tummy tuck. I'm still gutted I didn't get that!

I saw my hysterectomy as complete freedom. Freedom from the wretched periods every month, the pain every month, the bloating every month, the "have I got enough tampons and sanitary towels?" every month, the "ooh, I'd better not pack anything white, just in case I come-on when I'm away".

I was blissfully unaware of what to expect as time went on. I was starting to get to know my body without period pains etc., and the months and then years just ticked by. So, when I felt something that I hadn't felt before, I looked it up to see if it was possibly a menopausal symptom, found out what could naturally work, tried it, and 9 times out of 10 it worked. Was it really that simple? Honestly? For me, yes it was.

You know your body better than anyone else. I knew I wasn't ill, because I didn't feel ill. I just felt odd. When my body told me it needed or was lacking something, I listened. I researched what it could possibly be and found what I thought would help, what had helped other women around the world, and, as I said before, it worked! So now, I expect you would like to read some examples?

Before you look into thinking these will work for you, you MUST talk to your doctor first, especially if you're on any medication, as some supplements etc., can interfere with medication you've been prescribed. I would also strongly advise you go to your doctor first, if you're at all worried about anything, just in case it might be an underlying health condition and not connected to the menopause.

What worked for me, here we go...

❖ *Aches and pains,* I took glucosamine sulphate, and all my aches and pains went. I still take half a tablet every day.

❖ *Hair thinning* to the point that I wore a wig. I took 2 x sea kelp tablets a day and it all grew back, even better than before in fact. I still take 1 tablet a day.

❖ *Low mood*, I took vitamin D and my mood improved. I still take 1 tablet a day.

❖ *Anxiety* out of the blue! I took magnesium and vitamin B12 every day, and within a week, my anxiety had gone. I still take 1 tablet a day. I also took vitamin C, omega-3-fish-oil and a good quality multi-vitamin. All these helped too with my energy levels and mood. I still take these daily.

❖ *Osteoporosis* can be a problem as we get older. I take a calcium tablet every night.

❖ *Dry skin and wrinkles* (absolutely not, no, no, no), so I used coconut oil, every night and they softened to the point of disappearing.

❖ *Weight gain* (our metabolism slows down during menopause), so I ate smaller meals on a smaller plate. I chewed more, drank a glass of water before eating and only ate when I was hungry. This is something that I still do. I've noticed that I don't need anything like the quantity of food I did when I was younger.

Another good piece of advice I received was to "eat like a King for breakfast, a Queen for lunch and a Pauper for dinner", and don't eat too late at night. I did a home workout, only 15 minutes in the morning and lost over 1 stone in under 2 months. No equipment and no-one knew. I just got thinner and fitter and felt so much better. Also, power-walking is so good, not only for your mental health and your fitness levels, but also for your bones.

I did so much research over the years after my hysterectomy, that I created *The Secret Solutions to Menopause Symptoms*[1]. So I was busy, yes, and personally I think that really helped me through those early years, because I didn't have time to think about me. I suppose I became stronger than my body with controlling it, rather than it controlling me.

The girls grew up, they didn't need me as much as they used to and that's when everything changed. As a mother, you put everything and everyone first before yourself, and that's perfectly normal. But when the children grew up, what I wasn't prepared for was TIME. Will surgical menopause change you? Absolutely! So, try and use this time to change yourself in a good way, and it's something that every woman can do.

Who was I? I'd changed from the woman I was when I had the girls, but I didn't know who I was now. So that started the next and exciting chapter of my life. Time to start looking at ME. I needed to re-discover ME. The ME I wanted to become. I tried to look at it a bit like emerging from a chrysalis into a butterfly. I didn't want the menopause to master me, I was going to master the menopause and the years ahead of me.

Over the coming months, I changed my hair, my makeup, my wardrobe, some of my friends, my hobbies and interest, my skincare routines, my fitness, in fact my life. I changed so much and started to feel happier and look younger, that my friends started to comment and asked me to help them. I was told I should help other women by sharing what I'd done. And so, my social-media journey began, which was slightly hairy. At that time I'd only been able to master how the microwave and my phone worked. But, as they say, 'ignorance is bliss' and they're absolutely right.

If I'd overthought my hysterectomy and surgical menopause, I'm sure it would have been a lot harder. If I'd overthought "oh you just start a Facebook group[2]", or talking on Radio 1, or becoming an author[3], then chances are those things would have been much harder.

All that was in my 50's. What do they say? You're never too old, and they're absolutely right. Each one of us has so much to offer. The key is to grab the opportunities and run with them. Go whichever road they take you down, because if one door closes, it's because it's not meant to be your door and invariably another, much better door opens instead.

I hear from women in pain all over the world, women who just want their life back. They want to stop being in pain, feeling lost, scared, alone, or thinking they're going mad. Something had to be done. If we wait for doctors to care enough, for men to care enough, maybe even some of our friends to care enough, for the medical industry to care enough, we'll be waiting years and years and that's not right or fair! And so, in my 60's, frustrated with the status-quo, I embarked on another new venture and founded an online membership club[4]. It's a virtual space with menopause experts waiting to help you, where questions are answered, and where there is help and support available by the bucket load.

My parting advice would be, only follow sites and groups that are positive and helpful. See your surgical menopause as the start of a new journey and make this the most enjoyable, rewarding, satisfying time of your life, because being older is great, you can get away with so much more!

Love Shelley x

[1]*The Secret Solutions to Menopause Symptoms https://py.pl/1N5b4Z*
[2]*Closed Facebook Group*
https://www.facebook.com/groups/MenopauseHelp/
[3]*Menopause Matters – How to Master the Menopause, Survive, Thrive and Feel Alive*
http://amzn.eu/55VFZGF
[4]*Experts, Knowledge Centre, Lives, Articles, How to Guides, The Membership Club -*
which gives you access to everything and the Club Facebook Group
www.menopausehelp.org

Shelley (whose menopause journey made her into a butterfly) Chapman started helping friends through their menopause, and then someone set Shelley up on social media which she describes as "an interesting learning curve". Shelley now helps women all over the world transition through their menopause and beyond. A worldwide author and speaker, Shelley is driven by a passion to get her message across that we're never too old to discover a new life on the other side of menopause.

Chapter Nine

Emily Grace, 30

"I am thankful for my struggle, because without it I wouldn't have stumbled upon my strength."

- Alexandra Elle -

Growing up in the East Midlands, I was a happy, carefree child, with lots of friends and a loving family. I enjoyed school and was very active. Barely an evening passed where I didn't have some kind of extracurricular activity planned. My main passion was gymnastics, but I also enjoyed swimming, Brownies, dance, and I had a love for being outdoors. When I hit puberty I continued to be active, now having a preference for swimming, running and hockey. However, this was also around the time my journey with poor mental health began.

By the time I reached my teens, I experienced regular panic attacks and struggled with an eating disorder and self-harm. Despite my difficulties, I finished school with good grades, completed A levels and graduated from university with a 2:1 BSc in Physiotherapy. Regardless of my objective success I continued to be plagued with self-doubt and self-criticism and crippled by anxiety and depression, which manifested themselves through my anorexia and self-harm.

For years I took numerous psychiatric medications and attended hours of therapy, but there was never any significant lasting progress. Life seemed to be a revolving cycle of self-destruction, which sadly resulted in me walking away from my dream career only three short years after qualifying.

Too emotionally unstable and unwell to work, I did once question if my reproductive hormones could potentially be contributing to my poor mental health, but this issue was outright dismissed by the psychiatrist who said "wouldn't it be nice if it was it *just* hormones". I was young, naïve and vulnerable, I had my healthcare professionals on a pedestal and didn't dare pursue the issue any further.

It wasn't until I was sat shaking with anxiety, staring at the floor, that one day my GP had the courage to think outside the box and look beyond my pre-existing diagnostic labels. I remember that appointment vividly. I'd been seeing the same GP for some time, she was unlike any other medical professional I'd met. However bad things became, she always believed I had the strength to get past them.

Through my regular visits, she began to pick up on some patterns; how I always seemed to be at my worst the day before my period was due. One day I would be at rock bottom and the next day I felt out of the darkness again, and there had only been one change. During that 24-hour window I had come on my period, and with that my distress and despair would begin to dissipate. It was in that appointment that my GP told me she thought I had a condition called premenstrual dysphoric disorder (PMDD).

Initially I was sceptical, to me it just seemed like yet another diagnosis, surely there was no way that something as simple as a period could have this much impact? Over the years, I'd been tracking my menstrual cycle on a calendar and writing about my mental health on a blog and when I looked at the two side by side, I was floored. Every time my period was due, my mental health plummeted. Everything matched up. Clinging on to hope, and desperate for change, I was willing to explore every avenue. And thus begun my journey with gynaecology.

Prior to surgery I was a keen runner, having ran two marathons and more half marathons than I care to count. I still enjoy running although as you read my narrative you will find that it is a lot harder now.

I agreed to share my story and contribute to this book as my journey has made me passionate about raising the profile of both women's health and mental health. I work hard to reduce stigma, ensure people know their rights and have the most up to date, correct educational information and resources available, to enable them to make informed decisions about their own healthcare. I enjoy creating platforms for others to find their voice, speak out and to help them feel heard.

Why?

At the very beginning of this gynaecology journey, I had a perfectly healthy uterus, fallopian tubes and ovaries. You see for me, the problem wasn't my tissues. There was no history of heavy menstrual bleeding or any physical pain, and I was lucky not to have cysts, growths or any cancer. My ovaries were also in fine form, having produced just the right amount of hormones to regulate my body temperature, protect my heart health and keep my bones nice and strong. So why at the age of 28 and longing for a family was I counting down the days until I got a total hysterectomy? Because I was living with PMDD.

PMDD is a hormone-based mood disorder affecting around 1 in 20 females of reproductive age. The symptoms, which typically only occur between ovulation and menses, are largely psychological in nature, including: severe depression, anxiety and irritability, extreme mood swings, difficulty concentrating, fatigue, insomnia, and a feelings of being overwhelmed and out of control. These are often severe enough to cause a person to want to end their life rather than continue to experience them.

By definition PMDD is an abnormal reaction to a normal change in hormone levels across the menstrual cycle. As my oestrogen fell and my progesterone rose (as it's supposed to) each month, I became enveloped in depression, hopelessness and worthlessness, whilst simultaneously my anxiety levels would sky-rocket. I did anything, regardless of consequences, to make it stop. PMDD affects all aspects of life; your ability to work, study and maintain intimate relationships. Tragically, it is estimated that 30% of all PMDD sufferers will attempt to take their life. I was part of that statistic.

But why now? I'd battled mental health difficulties (anorexia nervosa, deliberate self-harm, depression & anxiety) for a number of years before seeking professional support at the age of 18. I had a medication history spanning the alphabet, and I'd received an incorrect label of emotionally unstable personality disorder (EUPD).

Despite being desperate for change, I struggled with therapists and "hoodwinked" members of the community mental health team into believing I was okay, only to have another crisis days later. I was told I was motivated, hardworking and very aware of my difficulties, yet it didn't seem to make any difference. Regardless of the support I was given I never seemed to make any real progress - until September 2016, when I was *finally* diagnosed with PMDD.

Slowly my life began to make sense and I realised that my mental health problems had begun right when I hit puberty, which coincidentally, is when hormones are surging and fluctuating at high intensity. By the time I started my periods, my difficulties had become full blown disorders. As the responsibilities of life increased, I struggled to simply keep up. I was constantly trying to repair the damage and feeling guilty for my actions and behaviours which had occurred during my PMDD episodes.

It was a never-ending cycle. Starvation numbed my emotions and helped me find control in a world where I felt completely out of control, but more than that, I believe it reduced the hormonal fluctuations. The deliberate self-harm led to the diagnosis of EUPD, yet I maintained my actions were all pre-meditated to cause as little disruption to my life as possible. I just needed a break from the unbearable distress of my own mind.

My illness resulted in multiple medical appointments each week, predominantly for my mental health, and for at least two weeks each month, twenty-four-hour supervision and support from family and friends. For the five years prior to surgery I wasn't able to work. The year before surgery I had a permanent inpatient bed at the local psychiatric unit as the risk to my life had become too great and it was impossible to keep me safe in the community. Life was far from "normal", but back then, it was my normal.

Choosing surgery

Following my diagnosis, I had tried a short period of unopposed addback oestrogen, which seemed to alleviate my anxieties somewhat, and then a few weeks later I was fitted with a Mirena coil. Unfortunately, this was promptly taken out due to adverse side effects. It wasn't long before my doctor realised that alongside PMDD, I was also severely progesterone intolerant. However, I was warned of the risks of using unopposed addback oestrogen.

It was in that same appointment, not far into my journey with gynaecology, that I first heard the words "*I think it is likely that this might result in a hysterectomy*". I left the room and walked down the long sterile hospital corridor before reaching a bench where myself and my mum sat down to process what I had just been told. I was 26 and I guess very naïve. I had a problem with my hormones, not my uterus. Surely I wouldn't need to have a hysterectomy?

The news hit my mum hard. Her little girl, who had always talked and dreamed of having children, had just been told she might need to have a hysterectomy and there was nothing she could do to fix it. As we sat on the bench, I remained strong and optimistic, comforting my mum and telling her everything was going to be okay as silent tears rolled down her face. Before long we got up, brushed ourselves off and worked out how we were going to break the news to the rest of the family. We drove home in silence, neither one of us daring to speak in case we said the wrong thing and upset the other again.

Fast forward two years and multiple gynaecology appointments. I had been referred to a specialist PMDD clinic where I was rapidly working my way through the PMDD treatment recommendations. I had been placed in an induced chemical menopause and tried multiple different preparations, doses, brands and duration of combined HRT, but we were fast running out of options.

Throughout this whole journey, there was only one thing that had given me any real lasting relief, a blissful trial of chemical menopause and oestrogen-only HRT. The doctor had called it a progesterone "holiday", a break from the treatment to simulate what life could be like if they were able to successfully eradicate the hormonal fluctuations which were occurring each month due to my menstrual cycle. It was honestly the best three months of my life. I didn't have a single down day.

In disbelief, I made a bucket list, determined to reclaim my life. They were minor things to most people, like going kayaking, watching a film at an outdoor cinema, being able to see my best friend graduate, eating at Planet Hollywood, seeing a West End Show, attending Bristol International Hot-Air Balloon Fiesta and visiting the Leaning Tower of Pisa. My friend and I booked a four-day trip to Italy. Despite planning to come home if my mental health should plummet, there wasn't a single difficult moment. Gazing up at the Leaning Tower of Pisa on my first holiday in five years, I breathed in the warm Italian air. Then and there, I decided that I couldn't go back to life as it was before, I wanted this feeling to last forever.

When I returned and spoke with my doctors, I was heartbroken to learn chemical menopause with oestrogen-only HRT wasn't a long-term solution because denying your body progesterone for an extended period of time can cause dangerous abnormal cell growth in the womb lining. However tough it was on me mentally, I had to start taking some progesterone again, and thus started my 11-month admission to the local psychiatric hospital.

Before long I was not only having to take progesterone, but the chemical menopause had also started to fail to fully suppress my menstrual cycle. It was then that the doctors told me I should seriously consider having a full hysterectomy, removing my uterus, fallopian tubes, both ovaries and my cervix. While less invasive methods work for many other people with PMDD, sadly I was in the small percentage who were classed as treatment-resistant and the only hope of safely finding long term relief was in the form of irreversible and potentially risky surgery.

Of course, I could just choose to keep my reproductive organs, but at what cost? Life often felt unbearable, my reproductive hormones were regularly throwing me into crisis, the anxiety overwhelming and the frustration and despair crushing. This wasn't like any usual emotional distress; it was intense and unrelenting.

Experiencing that level of emotional suffering month after month was exhausting and amid the inner turmoil my urge was always just to make it stop. I was insistent I didn't want to kill myself, yet time and time again found myself engaging in self destructive, often life threatening, and dysfunctional behaviours in order to try and find some relief from the symptoms.

During the periods of calm between the chaos I would frantically scramble to repair my life, to catch up on my seemingly never ending "to-do" list. I would burn the candle at both ends, my days long as I woke early and stayed up late, editing videos, baking cakes, hand crafting cards, raising awareness of PMDD, doing anything to escape my true reality. I would travel the country and cram in back-to-back visits to spend time with friends and family knowing that it was only a matter of days before I would be heading back into the darkness again.

It was exhausting. I was tired. But this wasn't any kind of tired though, this was a deeply depressed, 'I can't carry on like this much longer', kind of tired. I had reached my threshold of resilience. After years of what I can only describe as a living hell, I did not feel strong enough to keep going through this vicious cycle any longer.

A last resort

I was out of treatment options, but there was one thing I clung to that gave me a thread of hope - the option of surgery and a progesterone free life. At this point it was a choice between my future self, my life and my fertility. I didn't want to go on fighting for survival anymore. I was fully dependant on others, I didn't have a job and I was deemed too unstable to drive. With my ever-fluctuating mood I struggled with relationships and despite desperately wanting children, the reality of being stable enough to have a relationship and build a life outside of the hospital felt like a distant dream.

Then came the question of what would happen if I did have children? Current research points to PMDD having a genetic factor, so what if I somehow got myself stable and then passed this awful condition on to my children or grandchildren? I couldn't bear to watch them go through even half of what I had been through. Even if I had children, what sort of a mother would I be? As it stood, I couldn't care for myself let alone a child. I worried about the impact my illness would have on any potential offspring. I couldn't do it; it wouldn't be fair.

Every area of my life felt completely out of control. I feared that if I didn't make an informed decision to have surgery now, then in time that decision was going to be taken out of my hands. I had to be strong. In a life full of chaos and uncertainty there was one thing I could take control of, and that was my body.

I played out all the possible options for my future over and over in my mind for some months, and once I was clear about the decision I had made, I dared discuss it with family, friends and professionals. In coming to terms with it there were tears, so many tears and I vividly remember lying on my bed crying for days. The emotional pain was unimaginable, as if I had been winded. For so many years therapists had used my strong desire to have my own family as a tool to ground me, help me engage in therapy and give me a reason to live and yet now I was making the conscious decision to give up the one thing I had held on so long for. Somehow though, I felt a sense of peace with my decision.

Discussions with friends and professionals raised a lot of questions, predominantly, what if I regretted the surgery? Luckily, I was supported by a great team of professionals and after numerous discussions over many months, they knew I had explored all options, both long and short term, and were happy to back me in my decision. So, we went ahead and put in the application for surgery, but without an immediately evident, life threateningly unhealthy uterus or ovaries, little did I realise the challenges I would have finding a surgeon who would operate on a 29-year-old female who hadn't completed her family. However, many appointments, phone calls, tear stained tissues and months later, my case was taken to the gynaecology multidisciplinary team meeting and my decision was finally approved.

Being "young" and not having had any children yet, it was difficult to find any sort of literature on what my rights were with regards to fertility. All the protocols and papers discussed those undergoing treatment and surgery for cancers, but nothing for PMDD or any other conditions. Luckily, my fantastic GP raised the issue with the local NHS commissioning board (the organisation who funds NHS treatments) and in order to keep my options open, I was able to have one full round of fertility treatment for egg harvesting on the NHS.

Fertility prior to surgery was yet another emotional rollercoaster. Preparing my body to produce multiple eggs and suppress ovulation until after egg collection made me feel maternal and protective. Despite the ongoing emotional turmoil and urges to self-destruct, over and over I grounded myself. I knew I literally had one attempt at this. If I overdosed or significantly harmed myself now, I could mess this whole thing up and that would be my chances of future IVF via a surrogate gone. How would I feel about that? Would I forever grieve and feel guilty about it? Yes probably.

The process of the fertility treatment was terribly lonely, and it seemed everywhere I looked there were reminders of what I couldn't have - children! Sitting in the clinic I felt I was the only person alone, without a partner, instead sitting there with my mum whilst they took blood, did scans and worked out what treatment I needed next. Eventually, the treatment was all over, seventeen eggs were collected, and it was then just a matter of time until I got a date for my hysterectomy.

I was determined that instead of mourning my losses, I was going to celebrate the chance of a new life and a fresh start. The weekend before my hysterectomy, I got all my friends together and threw a hysterectomy party. Everyone wore pink, except for me, I wore a grey t-shirt emblazoned with *"See you later ovulator"*. One friend brought me a hospital survival kit complete with a stuffed "super uterus" and friends served my uterus "eviction letters" - notes of support to remind me why I had made this decision for me to read when feeling lonely in the hospital. There were red and pink coloured food and drinks, we played pin the egg on the uterus, and there was a uterus piñata, before finishing the evening off with shots of strawberry crème baileys through plastic syringes.

Surgery

My hysterectomy was booked for 7th May 2019. It was a gorgeous late spring day and I woke early, feeling galvanised and strong. I even filmed a vlog for my YouTube channel before we left for the hospital. This was going to be the first day of the rest of my life. But still, a seed of doubt niggled. Was I doing the right thing? What if it didn't work? Despite being the first patient on the afternoon list, it was a long morning of bubbling anticipation. I was visited by numerous doctors and nurses to talk over the plans for the procedure. As I had clinically healthy ovaries, I'd chosen to donate one to science, whilst the other would be retained as part of an Ovarian Tissue Cryopreservation Project (OTCP).

I had never had an operation before, so being wheeled down the hospital corridors into the anaesthetic room was a very surreal feeling. I recall being asked to sit on the edge of the bed with my knees up to my chest and bend forwards whilst they inserted the epidural. But on questioning, I could still feel my legs, so they repeated the procedure after which I quickly lost any sensation in my legs.

Lying on the trolley the doctor told me he was going to give me a sedative and then a general anaesthetic. I lay there thinking in a minute I will feel myself slowly drifting off or they will ask me to count down backwards from ten or something daft, but nothing. One minute we were chatting away and then I was gone. I am told the procedure lasted about two and a half hours, but between those final moments in the anaesthetic room to waking up with my parents beside me in a side room on the ward, I remember very little.

When I woke up I remember vividly the first thing I asked was how the surgery went. I had been told they planned to do a laparoscopically assisted vaginal hysterectomy (LAVH), removing everything through the vagina, but if required they might need to do open surgery. With my track record of failed treatment attempts, I half expected to find they'd needed to cut me open. However, to my surprise there were only four little incisions, each with a single dissolvable stitch: one above each hip, one near my pubic bone and one inside my belly button.

My recollection of that evening is very hazy. I could move my arms, but I still had no sensation to touch which became apparent when the nurse took blood and I didn't feel a thing. I still couldn't feel or move my legs, so getting out of bed to go to the toilet was not possible but thankfully I had a urinary catheter.

That evening I was taught how to give myself an injection (into my stomach) of an anti-coagulant to help prevent blood clots. I would need to do this every day for the next two weeks. Having just undergone major surgery I was advised I would need lots of rest and that my movement was likely to be quite limited for the first few weeks.

At 8pm my visitors were asked to leave. I was left alone laying in the side room, totally immobile and feeling empty, with a call bell in close reach, staring at the same three, bare, blank walls. Thank goodness for my phone and headphones because I had a long night ahead of me. Routing through my overnight bag I found a card which my mum had left for me. We are big music lovers in our family and inside was a playlist of inspirational and motivational songs. It was such a magical idea and knowing my family had picked out these anthems based on the lyrics of each song helped soothe me no end.

The following morning was busy. I was seen by the doctor on his ward round and informed everything had gone well. I had my catheter removed and I was also seen by the physiotherapist who gave me some exercises I could do at home to help strengthen my pelvic region. There was just one issue, I still couldn't properly feel my torso or my legs. It was as if the messages were getting blocked. If I thought about wriggling my toes or moving my legs, the action happened almost in slow motion and any feedback from my limbs to my brain was limited and delayed. Having some background experience of working in healthcare, I was confident this was just the aftereffects of the anaesthetic and epidural which hadn't yet worn off. I just needed time.

But the response from some of the staff troubled me as they demanded I just stand up and walk to the toilet. I felt small and bewildered. I was sure they couldn't have received a full hand-over and were judging me on my age, and the fact I didn't have cancer and were therefore assuming I must just have had a little investigative procedure.

Fortunately, I was able to make my voice heard, a bladder scan was done and a catheter reinserted to drain my, by now, very full bladder. You see, I had enough sensation to know that I wanted to wee, but I hadn't yet regained enough sensation or control back over my muscles to actually be able to go to the toilet. It felt like torture.

Luckily, soon enough the sensation did return and the following day I felt like a new woman. I was able to go to the toilet on my own. I showered, put on clean clothes and even went for a few walks down the corridor and outside to get some fresh air. Just over 48 hours after I had been admitted, I was pain free and on my way home. Initially there were a number of precautions I had to follow, no lifting anything heavier than a kettle for six weeks. I could walk, but no running, no swimming, no vigorous activity, and no sex.

In the days that followed my surgery I was incredibly lucky, I had no bleeding. I remained pain free throughout, but I did a lot of sleeping. My stomach area remained bloated for several days, if not weeks, from the swelling and the gases they pumped into me to create room to move my organs around during the surgery. After a few days I dared to peel back the small gauzes and look at my wounds, neat and tidy but very bruised.

Life post-op

My ovaries, the reason for the distress caused by the hormonal fluctuations throughout my menstrual cycle, were gone, but what did that really mean for me and the rest of my life? Was I now "fixed", rendering the notion that prior to this I had somehow been a broken version of myself?

Despite anecdotal warnings from others that it would take some months, if not a couple of years for my hormones to stabilise post-op, from a medical standpoint it certainly did seem as if there was very little consideration given to all the emotional trauma my experiences of life up to that point had left me with.

Spending 11 months as an inpatient on an acute psychiatric ward, the nurses had become a bit like a second family to me. They had seen me in some of the darkest moments, they had provided distractions and safety in moments of physical and emotional distress. Being on the ward as I went through my fertility journey, inadvertently they had been beside me in that too. They had watched the rise and fall of my emotional turmoil every month and had been with me on the countdown to my surgery day. In the better times we had laughed and joked and danced around the ward, it wasn't all terrible, there were some good memories too.

For all that time I had been fortunate enough to have 24-hour, 7-day support from professionals and family and yet less than a week after life changing surgery I felt that all my support was gone. I didn't know what life post-op was going to look like for me, and yet I was discharged from both the medical and the psychiatric hospital and the care of the crisis team and community mental health nurses.

All I was left with was a psychiatrist who I had never met and wouldn't meet for another 6 months, GP follow up as and when I booked in, an hour slot each fortnight with the psychologist, and an 8-week post-op check with the consultant. There was no menopause clinic follow up, no women's health or pelvic physio appointments. Nothing. Just a big wide void. I was free and it was simultaneously amazing and terrifyingly daunting.

I had been so used to living a "half-life", what did I now do with all this free time?! I began to realise that over the years my entire identity had been bound up in illness. If I wasn't ill with my eating disorder, then it was self-harm, overdoses or PMDD. So, if the cause of all that had been removed, then who was I now?

My mood on any given day would determine how I answered that question. Some days the world was my oyster, I was motivated and eager to do my little bit to change the way others were treated. I felt optimistic and strong. I was no longer tied down with the burden and heaviness of PMDD and I could achieve anything I set my mind to. I was so lucky, almost 30 years old and a complete blank canvas to create whatever vision of myself and life I wanted to choose for my future.

Other days life felt much bleaker as I ruminated on all the years I had lost to PMDD. I grieved my abandoned career, the many broken relationships, both romantic and other, and for the children I would never bare. Without the constant love and support from friends and family it could have been so easy to give up on life and slide back into a terribly deep dark depression.

Whilst having a fresh start could be exciting, at times it was also incredibly overwhelming. Where did I even start with getting my life on track? All around me friends were getting married and having children, yet I didn't even have a job, let alone a stable relationship or any prospects of being able to provide for a family anytime soon. I felt a sense of crushing failure, my life was a mess!

The weeks that followed were mixed. Everything had changed, and nothing had changed all at once. Although my future looked a little different now, I was still the same Emily, but having just undergone major surgery, I was somewhat taken aback by the reaction of friends and family. It seemed that my hysterectomy was the elephant in the room. Everyone knew it had happened, but no one dared to ask me how I was for fear of upsetting me.

Once again I felt so alone, like I didn't matter and no one cared. Of course, the reality was very far from that made-up truth my mind had created. The reason everyone was avoiding asking the obvious question was fear. Fear of upsetting me and perhaps fear of hearing replies which would make them feel uncomfortable, or to which they didn't know how to respond.

From a physical standpoint, my swelling began to dissipate and slowly the initial post-op fatigue began to pass. But what remained was a significant weakness around my pelvic region. Having once been a keen runner, I was now struggling to walk, stand or sit for any prolonged period. My core felt so weak and an ache around my hips and deep within my back would soon develop which forced me to sit or lay down with my back supported in order to find some relief.

Despite there being no pain from the surgery itself, the physical recovery was a lot slower than I anticipated, however I did eventually get back to running again. I was slow as hell and seriously out of practice, but at least I got out there and had a go. As a result of an online group called "Running through menopause", I met a wonderful network of people who were in a similar position to myself.

Having been in chemical menopause and on HRT prior to surgery, I figured out that luckily I had already done my crash course in hormone health and I was well prepared for the problems that I may face with my hormones when my body was thrown into surgical menopause. I was also fortunate to be a part of numerous Facebook support groups for individuals who'd undergone surgery as final stage treatment for their own treatment-resistant PMDD and hormone sensitivity, so I thought I knew what to expect. However, despite having read of the struggles others faced trying to get their hormone levels 'right' post op, I was convinced I would be the exception. Surely I had endured my fair share of problems already, after all nothing could be worse than living a minute longer with PMDD!

They say 'forewarned is forearmed' and so with the knowledge that it may take 18 months to 2 years for my hormones to stabilise post-op (although initially not wanting to admit that things were becoming tough again) it came as no surprise to me when, after a few weeks of relative emotional bliss, I noticed a resurgence of poor mental health. My mood plummeted and my brain went on autopilot as the urges to self-destruct returned.

Only now things were so different. There was space to stand back and breathe, space to process my thoughts and what was happening. Despite the urges feeling overwhelming at times, I knew I didn't want to engage in them. The impulsivity that for me came coupled with hormone fluctuations and PMDD was gone! After all those years, although my body was still seemingly doing strange things with my hormones, and in turn my emotions, I finally felt in control of my actions. Despite struggling with my mental health for all my teenage and adult life, now amidst the urges and the depression, I felt calm, this was a new feeling for me. I wasn't really sure what was happening, but I labelled it as "normal" depression, if there were ever such a thing! No longer fighting for survival each day, I became filled with feelings of boredom and hopelessness. What was the point in life? I found it difficult to find a reason to peel myself out of bed and shower each morning. I knew something wasn't right and I guessed the answer lay in my hormone levels.

However, discharged from the surgeon at 8 weeks post op with my wounds healing well and no immediate concerns, I had no further follow up planned. So, I took it upon myself to continue fighting for my health as I had done for all those years before. I booked myself in to discuss my concerns with my GP who was very amenable to carrying out blood work to find out just what my hormone levels were doing.

My GP and I were muddling through. I was an expert in knowing how I felt and my GP was excellent at knowing her job, but neither of us were hormone or menopause specialists. Although my hormone levels fell within what was classed as normal/acceptable for a menopausal woman, I knew my body and I was convinced something wasn't right. I was fairly sure that 'something' was my hormone levels.

I immediately tried to get myself booked into a local menopause clinic for follow up, only to find that the specialist consultant had recently left, there was no replacement and waiting times were lengthy. I was frustrated and angry. I had lived a half-life for far too long. I hadn't been through all of this and given up my fertility to continue to live in a fog of hormonal hell all because no one could advise me if my current HRT regime was still adequate. I wasn't prepared to sit back and wait. To them I might have just been another statistic on a waiting list, but this was MY LIFE!

I wasted no time in arranging for a private consultation where the doctor explained that she was not surprised I was feeling so dreadful. Yes, my levels were within normal range for a menopausal woman, but I wasn't experiencing a normal menopause. I was not yet 30, my oestrogen needs were much greater than someone in their 50's or 60's. The specialist advised on what oestrogen levels we should be aiming for, my HRT prescription was altered and within days I was a changed woman, confident, enthusiastic, and motivated once again.

Now equipped with the information needed to move forwards, although not always advisable, guided by my subjective experience of symptoms, over the coming months myself and my GP monitored my blood hormone levels on a number of occasions, and I underwent HRT adjustments to help stabilise my hormones within an acceptable range. Finally, we seemed to have reached a plateau. Life was good. I continued to see a psychologist to help me work through some of the finer details of adjusting to my new life back at home but there were no more crises or hospital admissions. By now I was 6 months post-op and getting itchy feet. I had waited for this level of stability in my life for so long and I was eager to move on and leave my life with PMDD behind me. November 2019 was a whirlwind month for me. Despite my GP and psychologist advising me to take it slow, to take time to heal emotionally and to adapt to my new life, I decided I was done with waiting.

Within a month, I'd moved house, applied for and secured a job in healthcare, brought a car, got my license back and turned 30. Naively I honestly thought that was where my story would end. My hormones were stable, I had my new life, now all I had to do was live it. If only that had been how things turned out for me, but unfortunately it wasn't.

Just weeks into finally being stable and feeling everything was sorted, the nationwide UK HRT shortage kicked in and I had to switch from patches to gels. What an absolute nightmare! You see, although all HRT gives you the same end result, there can be considerable individual variation in efficacy between different products. As I switched from patches to gels, it took time for my body to adjust. The location of absorption had also changed, so this resulted in yet more hormone fluctuations.

However, it didn't end there, and we struggled to get my oestrogen levels back within the desired range.

After yet another 2 months of hormonal mood disruption and now 8 months post-op, I was finally back under a specialist and my HRT prescription was changed again. I started a new job and at last I was feeling well in myself again. However before long, I was coming home exhausted, experiencing frequent migraines, having multiple hot flushes a day and despite the overwhelming fatigue my sleep was constantly being disturbed with vivid dreams and regular night sweats.

In spite of all this there was one positive, my mood felt more stable than ever before. I was coping at work, in fact I was doing more than coping, I was thriving both in my paid employment and in my voluntary roles. I was using my lived experience to increase awareness and hopefully improve things for others. I was invited to speak on BBC national news, my story was published in Cosmopolitan magazine and I was working with several professionals to raise the profile of PMDD.

For months, I chose to ignore the physical signs my body was giving me that something wasn't right. Regular migraines, feeling sapped of energy and poor temperature regulation were tough, but I would take those symptoms a million times over PMDD. These were the common symptoms of menopause I heard everyone speak about, and therefore I simply assumed feeling this way must be normal after a hysterectomy. I figured these symptoms were just something I needed to get used to and carried on the best I could.

Nonetheless before long the physical symptoms began to take their toll on my emotional health. My work-life balance was becoming more stretched each week and I found the all too familiar signs of depression and dread creeping back into my life. It was this dip in my mood and a sudden onset of panic coupled with exhaustion that prompted me to go back to visit my GP. Various blood work showed my oestrogen levels were too high and it became evident that despite my dose of HRT remaining constant for a number of months, I had developed oestrogen tachyphylaxis. We were then faced with the arduous task of bringing my oestrogen levels back down. This took a number of weeks if not months, but in time my blood hormone levels were finally back in range and I was able to start living again.

No longer fighting the physical side effects of surgical menopause and oestrogen tachyphylaxis, I was left with more free time and thinking space than ever before. My focus shifted to beginning to work on processing all I had been through and repairing my self-worth and self-confidence. I couldn't control every variable around me, but I was in charge of the value I placed on myself and my time, and how I chose to internalise or react to any given situation, enabling me to dictate the direction of my life from here on in.

However, despite this insight and a new positive outlook on life I know there are still hurdles to overcome. I still feel I am not yet the person I was supposed to be. I feel robbed of so much including my teenage years, the socially accepted transition into adulthood and my career, but most of all my ability to naturally conceive and carry my own child.

There is no escaping the reality, despite surgery eradicating the distress and dysfunction that came with my PMDD, the effects of the last 17 years, surgical menopause and hormone sensitivity will remain with me for life. Nevertheless, regardless of the challenges surgical menopause has brought me, I will never regret my surgery. I firmly believe it saved my life.

My tips for navigating surgical menopause include:

- A hysterectomy is major surgery. Following the operation, you may not be in pain and you may feel fine but it's important to follow post-op instructions. If, like me you had your hysterectomy performed laparoscopically, it might not look like you have many external wounds, but a lot happened internally.
- Don't suffer unnecessarily. If you are noticing a return of menopausal symptoms, then get things checked out, your HRT may need to be adjusted.
- Don't be afraid or ashamed to seek help and support for your emotional wellbeing and mental health, you may experience a sense of grief and loss following surgery.
- Find the strength and courage to become your own advocate. Doctors are the experts in their field of medicine, but you are the only person who has lived your life and is an expert in you!
- Unless advised otherwise, always leave 6-8 weeks between HRT changes to allow your body time to adapt to the new dose and method of delivery.
- Never underestimate the power of reproductive hormones.
- Surgical menopause can often feel like a rollercoaster of physical and emotional symptoms. This is not pleasant, but it is quite common. Give yourself time to adjust and heal. Life does get better.
- You are not alone. Reach out and find support from others in a similar situation. A great source for me has been The Surmeno Connection[1] and also The Daisy Network[2].

Don't be ashamed of your story because you just might inspire or help someone going through the same things. Everyone will experience life with circumstances that may or may not be within their control. What we learn from these experiences helps to create who we are.

"Dear Past, thanks for the lesson. Dear Future, I am ready!"

[1]*www.thesurmenoconnection.com*
[2]*www.daisynetwork.org*

Emily currently works as an Occupational Therapy Support Worker in an acute medical hospital. She is also a volunteer and ambassador for her local Mental Health and Specialised Eating Disorder Organisation (First Steps ED) where for the last year she has been the Patient Public Involvement and Engagement (PPIE) Chair and adult lead. Following her own illness, Emily became a Trustee of The National Association for Premenstrual Syndromes (NAPS). Emily is a patient representative with the Royal College of Psychiatrists, and she is involved in several NHS England projects relevant to her own lived experiences of healthcare as a Patient and Public Voice (PPV) Expert Advisor.

Emily tweets as: @PeriodsPower

Chapter Ten

Donna Klassen, 53

Pre-surgery

In April of 2019, I discovered a lump in my right breast. It seemed to pop out of nowhere, although I had a strange, almost prescient feeling about breast cancer and had been doing breast exams more often than usual. Breast cancer is all around us, including in some people very close to me, and while most often I would think I would not be the one to get it, sometimes I would say "but why not me?"

The lump I found was close to the skin. It was not like anything I'd felt before. "What the hell is that?" I thought. My pulse quickened. "Holy Mother of God!". I could see a tiny puckering of the skin and looking back, I think I knew that it was breast cancer.

I spent the next 2 hours examining every inch of both breasts trying to make sense of what was happening. Even though the lump did not feel like anything I'd ever known, I decided that maybe it could be benign. I'm not sure if it was full-on denial or just my optimism as I am generally a "glass is half-full" type of person.

I decided I wouldn't google breast cancer types, only benign lumps. I learned about all of the different types of benign findings in breasts, despite that lingering feeling that my lump was breast cancer. Later that night I told my husband about the lump I'd found, but assured him it was nothing. I am a Licensed Clinical Social Worker (LCSW), so I practiced the techniques I recommend to clients. I caught myself when I was catastrophising and going to the worst-case scenario. Until you know something to be true, I know that worrying is not helpful. Luckily, I am also someone who can block things out. Denial is sometimes a useful tool!

I focused on work and didn't allow myself to think that I had breast cancer, despite the occasional touches of my breast that reminded me of the unusual lump. Falling asleep was harder, as I would touch that lump, looking for it to get smaller but knowing it wasn't.

Looking back, I'm surprised that I didn't figure out a way to get an immediate mammogram and sonogram. Instead, I made an appointment with my GP and he told me it was probably nothing. Whew. But I still had a nagging feeling and I followed up with the referral for the mammogram and ultrasound. Once there, I watched on the screen as the ultrasound was administered and even I could see there was something irregular about the shape of my own uninvited lump. I quickly looked to read the face of the technician and knew there was cause for concern. Later, the doctor came in to tell me that what they found was suspicious, and she squeezed me into a biopsy appointment 2 days later. That was another bad sign.

I was told it would take 5 days to get my results. I know that waiting is always the hardest part -- and is that ever true. Those were long, tortured days filled with a new Google search topic: types of breast cancer.

The doctor called with my results while I was at work. "I'm really sorry to tell you," he began but I don't remember hearing him finish the sentence. "Fuck, fuck, fuck. FUCK!" is how I responded to hearing the news that my biopsy confirmed I had breast cancer. I immediately left the building where I work in Manhattan and began walking down the street. I had no idea where I was going, or even why I was going, but I *had to* move.

I texted my colleagues to let them know why I left so suddenly. I then texted my husband and we began walking towards one another. We walked toward the clinic where I had the biopsy and picked up the results. I have breast cancer. Intraductal carcinoma. I have cancer. Fuck, fuck, fuck. OK. OK. OK.

Many appointments, many new doctors, and many decisions followed. Difficult conversations were had -- the most emotional were telling my four daughters and then my mother. My husband helped me throughout. After further tests and some suspicious spots in my other breasts, I decided on a DIEP flap double mastectomy procedure in which fat and veins from my abdomen would be removed and used to reconstruct my breasts. I felt good about my decision. I joked with friends and family about getting a "tummy tuck" and how I had "just enough fat", according to my plastic surgeon. Looking back, I realise that I have my mother's optimism and hopefulness, and how much this helped me get through these challenging times.

As part of the normal pre-op, the plastic surgeon ordered a magnetic resonance angiography (MRA) of my abdomen. A few days later, the surgeon called to say I needed to see a gynaecological oncologist, and that it was urgent.

Wait... *what*?

She went on to explain that the MRA picked up several large, concerning cysts on my ovaries. My ovaries? Wait… I'm getting ready for a double-mastectomy. Why are my ovaries suddenly a part of this conversation? I saw yet another new doctor, the gynaecological oncologist who told me the cysts in my ovaries were larger than six centimetre's and one contained an internal mass. I knew that "internal mass" was not a good thing. He said I would need to have my ovaries removed and should do so prior to the upcoming mastectomy.

I was stunned… fully not processing.

I had wrapped my head around the first surgery, feeling surprisingly no overly strong allegiance to my breasts, but this news was harder to take. Maybe it was just one surgery too far or perhaps as a mother I was unprepared for this loss. Something about this news pushed me further than my optimism signed up for. Even though I was deep into peri-menopause at my age, I was a mess.

It was explained to me that removing my ovaries was a "good thing" in relation to the breast cancer, that my particular cancer was fed by oestrogen so removing them would help starve out any cancer cells that may have spread. I was fuzzy and still not processing. *These are my ovaries*. Losing them meant immediate menopause. It seemed an undeniable altering of myself. I felt it would leave me shrivelled and old and less female. Post-menopausal. I cannot explain it, but the thought of having my ovaries removed levelled me more than my upcoming double mastectomy, which was now just 2 weeks away.

I remained in a haze, still not fully accepting why I needed the surgery, and easily reduced to tears. I was fighting the oophorectomy. What kind of name is that, anyway? It sounds like something an oompa-loompa would need. And the unspoken fear underneath it all was undeniable: it could be more cancer. This was the worst week of all. I still don't remember large parts of it.

Because the oophorectomy was a laparoscopic procedure, my team of doctors agreed I could have it a week before the 9-hour double mastectomy and reconstruction surgery. Why not merge them into one recovery? The night before the oophorectomy was the saddest for me, holding my husband and crying, knowing that things would be different. I went to the hospital with a heavy heart, and was tearful as they put me under. For whatever reason, a week later I went into the mastectomy with far more optimism and acceptance, even laughing as I was being prepared for the mastectomy. Luckily, the biopsy from the oophorectomy revealed I did not have ovarian cancer. I was relieved.

Post-surgery

After the mastectomy surgery, I woke to find myself insulated in puffy clouds of heat. Literally. I was padded, almost cocooned, in a medical hot bubble wrap of sorts. This was to protect the blood flood in my new breast veins (that were previously in my abdomen). Welcome to radical menopause! Holy suffocating heat. My hot flushes started and have yet to leave me.

I had heard it was common in surgical menopause to get the symptoms in a more intense way. Those rumours were not wrong.

My hot flushes feel like they start deep inside my abdomen, and then blaze up my body to my head. My face turns purple-red and the sweat is sop-able. Once home from the hospital, I parked myself in front of the air conditioner. I even slept there, or tried to as my sleep was super disrupted and not just from surgical recovery. You can't sleep through a hot flush!

The sleeplessness made everything more challenging. After a while, I decided not to perseverate on the negative feelings about my hot flushes. I felt I had exhausted my family's patience in complaining about them. In my mind, I worked to reframe it, to tell myself it's just a hot flush, it's normal, it will be over in a few minutes. I stopped making it a big deal. I actively adjusted.

But then there was another whammy. I knew I had to go on medication (anastrozole) to treat my oestrogen positive breast cancer, but I'd not focused on that yet. However, I started researching anastrozole, which was an aromatase inhibitor. It slowly dawned on me that this pill, would take away any remaining oestrogen. I would have NO oestrogen at all.

Just like how the oophorectomy was part of my treatment for breast cancer, the anastrozole works to oestrogen-starve any fly-away breast cancer cells that may be hiding somewhere (at least that's my understanding). That's a good thing, of course. Not doing so could mean stage IV, metastatic breast cancer later on. But I was still uneasy about taking anastrozole. There's a lot of debate about how long patients should stay on it, but the consensus is at least 5 years, but maybe even 7 to 10 years. That's a long time. I started reading about anastrozole and the other aromatase inhibitors in online breast cancer forums. I don't recommend doing that.

I knew that I did not have to start taking it immediately as I was still in recovery from the surgeries, but picked up the prescription anyway. I was waiting for a baseline bone scan before I started, as many women have major bone loss and osteoporosis, but I decided to take one tablet. I was worried that the longer I waited, the harder it would be to start. How can such a tiny pill hold such large consequences?

Well, this tiny pill is powerful. I awoke in the middle of the night to a reality I had never experienced before, both lips dried to my teeth and my tongue did not have an ounce of liquid in it. My mouth was sandpaper.

I was freaked out and did not take another dose for another few weeks. The idea of living in a body with no oestrogen didn't sound right. It's not normal, is it? I grew more and more ambivalent about starting on anastrozole, worried about how it would affect me. I became anxious about increased joint pain and stiffness, a perimenopausal symptom I had already been experiencing for the past 3 years. I dug in my heels, in denial about what I had to do. It was like I was having an adult temper tantrum regarding this course of treatment. No! I don't want to!

I spent the next 2 weeks reading more about the drug, especially comments made by other breast cancer patients. I ultimately focused on the more positive comments and decided that I needed to do it. I want to live a long life, one in which I know my (yet to be born) grandchildren. In the end I couldn't deny the facts directly in front of me, so I accepted the negative side effects in exchange for Life. I started to take the anastrozole and have not missed a dose since. When I take the pill, I tell myself that it is to stop the cancer from coming back. Acceptance.

Menopause Max

For me, it's hard to know how surgical menopause impacted me, because only 2 months later I was on anastrozole and in "menopause max" as I like to call being post-menopausal on an aromatase inhibitor. I don't know what my surgical menopausal experience would have been otherwise.

My worst symptom, one that I didn't expect, was that I grew indescribably hungry all the time, and in 3 months put on 10 pounds. My metabolism had come to a screeching halt. My body, already altered in shape from radical surgery, was thickening in new and uncomfortable places. Whose body *is* this? If I wasn't eating, I was thinking about eating, and this was absolutely new to me. This made me frustrated, especially because I had been encouraged to watch my weight as a tool to treat the cancer. Why couldn't I get this under control? I was always hungry and never full, regardless of what or how much I ate. I'd read that visceral fat can produce oestrogen. Was my body trying to beat the effects of the anastrozole? Was it going crazy trying to produce its own oestrogen? It was demoralising to be unable to rein myself in and an uncomfortable symptom, to say the least.

Another persistent issue was difficulty sleeping. This makes everything worse. I had heard of restless leg syndrome, but I was experiencing something similar but across my entire body. There was a certain tension that kept me from sleeping. I could not coax my muscles into relaxed mode. It routinely took me more than two hours to fall asleep, and then the hot flushes would wake me every hour. Maddening.

I returned to work full-time soon after my surgeries but could not combat the subsequent change in my focus, alertness and mood. I was fuzzy. Put simply, I did not feel like my former self, something seismic had shifted. I was doing my best to put on a good face, but my colleagues noticed the change, and that made me feel worse. Working in an intense environment, a day program for women experiencing acute postpartum depression and anxiety, I found myself tearful, exhausted, overwhelmed, irritable and forgetful. And always hungry. This was not a good combination when I had a job that required calm, focus and high energy. I found myself behaving more rashly than before, which was unlike me, and I lost my ability to self-regulate. I was just so tired. I would come home from work and dive into bed, barely able to talk to my family.

Then it became clear to me that I could no longer work at the same pace with the same job I had before all of this happened. It was just too much. I had a job where I was responsible for high-risk patients, and my symptoms were getting in the way of me being effective. We always talked to our pregnant and postpartum women about the importance of self-care and self-compassion. I was not practicing what I was preaching.

Ultimately, I had to accept that I needed more help and that many things, including my work life, also needed a reboot. I left my full-time job and decided to return to private practice. I feel lucky that I had these options, but it was painful.

I began working with a psychiatrist and a therapist. My psychiatrist, who works solely with women who have breast cancer, put me on Pristiq (an SNRI antidepressant), and that helps with my symptoms of irritability and tearfulness. I also started taking Gabapentin which aids my sleep. It's also thought to help with hot flushes.

However, more importantly, my psychiatrist made me feel okay about having to take these medications. I'm grateful that I have something to combat the effects of no oestrogen on my mental health. With my therapist, I talked about my frustration with my symptoms and wanting to just be back to my "normal" self. I was forced to look at myself as someone who needed help, not just someone who helps others. But most of all, we talked about acceptance. I had to fully accept that I am someone who is post-menopausal, and that I take anti-hormonal therapy that helps to stop the breast cancer from returning but also requires me to work harder to function at my new normal. Acceptance is not giving up, it's accepting where you are in the present moment fully and completely, and not fighting what has happened in the past. It was hard to do.

It's important to note how much I benefited from working in mental health throughout this cancer-menopause experience. The symptoms of postpartum depression are similar to the hormone induced changes in oestrogen that menopausal women face: irritability, tearfulness, difficulty concentrating, fatigue. Knowing this, I realised how menopausal women are also at high risk for these symptoms, and how I was one of these people. I believe it is why I was able to accept taking medications and going to therapy quickly, seeing first-hand how both can really help people.

I am also grateful that I have access to quality care in New York City. I found a physical therapist who specialises in treating breast cancer patients to help with the frozen shoulder I experienced after the mastectomy. I started seeing a new gynaecologist who also specialises in breast cancer patients and was prescribed hyaluronic acid for vaginal dryness. I needed this army of professionals to help me recover. I knew I had to take better care of myself, so I stopped telling myself I was too busy and I made the time to eat better and exercise. I reminded myself that I needed to accept my new normal instead of fighting it. I had to adapt.

Despite the onslaught of these symptoms of menopause, I also felt some relief. Before, the idea of being in menopause was intimidating. Now, I was *living* the change rather than anticipating it. However, despite having an amazing treatment team for breast cancer and the ovarian cysts, it would have been helpful if my doctors had been more complete in telling me what to expect with menopause in general and in my case, surgical menopause and going on anastrozole. Vaginal dryness? Irritability? Painful sex? Foggy thinking? These are caused by hormonal changes, rooted in biology & chemistry, so why did my doctors not discuss it with me? Science shouldn't be taboo. Surgical menopause is intense, like dropping off a cliff. Being on an aromatase inhibitor is 'menopause max', yet there was no preparation from my doctors. There should be more support and far less stigma in how doctors discuss it with their patients.

After my many surgeries, doctors wanted to know how my body was recovering (in relationship to the particular surgeries) but no one actually spoke to me about *how I was*. In speaking to friends, I heard similar stories and was surprised by the paucity of information and support regarding how menopause affects women's physical and mental health. This led me to co-found *Let's Talk Menopause*, a non-profit organisation designed to bring more attention to the symptoms and stages of menopause, so women have the information they need. The mission of *Let's Talk Menopause* is to create a world invested in women's health and wellness throughout menopause by advocating for better health care for women and ending the stigma around menopause.

At the end of this journey, I discovered some unexpected silver linings. It's freeing to be on the other side of menopause. It's oddly liberating. I'm finding being in my fifties exciting. It feels like a good place to pause and consider what I want to achieve next. I'm more confident in the person I am, more accepting of my flaws but far more certain of my strengths. I feel more creative and optimistic about my future. Time has more value than ever before.

Website: https://www.letstalkmenopause.org
Email: info@letstalkmenopause.org
Twitter: @LTMenopause

Donna Tweets at: @dklassentherapy

Chapter Eleven

Emma Skeates, 53

I was put into surgical menopause aged 44 due to an exceptionally high CA125 count, which just happens to be the antigen in your blood that acts as a tumour marker for ovarian cancer. Although I did NOT have this terrible silent killer, as the level was slowly rising it was seen as "sensible" to have the op and basically whip everything out with it.

Initially, I was nervous, I had been warned that the chances were the operation would be open abdominal surgery with a small possibility that it could be done laparoscopically. I was also warned that as I awoke from my anaesthetic, I would be a menopausal woman instantly. But, hey, what were my choices? Dreading every blood test and the threat of cancer or this? To me and my surgeon it was a no-brainer. I will make you laugh a little with my arrival into hospital which may well explain my post-op condition and tendency to be a tad "accident prone"

I was admitted into Worthing Hospital. I arrived for my scheduled hysterectomy to be confronted with a plastic cup. My premature elation that they were putting me straight onto that fabulous "dancing on the ceiling" medication was somewhat subdued when I was asked to provide a "sample" to ensure that I was not in fact 'with child' which could have been a nasty surprise for us all, child included!

Into the loo I dutifully went and filled up the little cup. How do people judge these things, I needed a 2-litre coke bottle! I put it on the bin whilst I got me draws back up. Washed my hands like a good girl, then used the super hygienic pull-paper to dry off the ol' mits and then stepped decisively on the foot operated bin whose lid of course, as it should, flew upwards, sending my entire wee sample flying up the wall and all over my new tunic.

Oh dear god, why me? So, I go to flush the loo again to try and get the old juices going so I can produce another sample and very quickly discover that I have in fact pulled the panic alarm and within seconds I was surrounded by nurses, porters, one junior doctor and my husband. Not in any true distress just staring aimlessly at my somewhat tasteless artwork all over the loo wall and desperately trying to pretend that I was soaked because of an over vigorous tap. Totally convinced I had got away with my latest misdemeanour, I threw back my pee covered hair and waltzed off to my bed with my sizeable derriere on full display as I'd forgotten to tie up the back of my gown. Let me tell you, glamour and dignity are overrated.

So, there it was, my entrance into hospital. My exit was not dissimilar as I got a round of applause on my departure. I have to tell you that my recovery from what WAS in the end a laparoscopic procedure, was an absolute breeze. I was told to "take it easy" for a few weeks as quite a lot of internal work had been done which was not seen from the outside and the pain relief I was on masked this trauma. So, with no further ado, I told my husband and children that no housework or "Mummy duties" were to be carried out for at least 18 months and that was that! They bought that for at least a week then realised they had been duped.

I was started on oestrogen patches immediately as I was seen as rather young to be plunged into full menopause but sadly, I was allergic to the plastic, so I was instantly put onto 2mg of oestrogen orally. This helped tremendously and although I found myself tearful and rather anxious from time to time, I didn't experience any hot flushes or aches and pains.

It was around this time that I started to write my blog[1] as I had noticed that my moods were all over the place and that I felt a sense of sadness that my days of fertility were over and that I had entered a period that most women that had gone before me would see as "the end of days". As I was a rather accident-prone character anyway, the blog made me realise that so many of my symptoms were actually rather amusing and the blog quickly took off as the funny side of the menopause. Before I knew it, I had over 150K followers and had found not only a way for ME to cope but for others too.

I think what the blog highlighted to me, was the total lack of meaningful and helpful information out there for women such as myself. I was inundated with messages about where to go, who to talk to, were the strangest symptoms actually menopausal or just individual. It was quickly evident to me that help was desperately needed for SO many women. I found my help in a group of doctors called The Menopause Consultancy[2] who I had a 45-minute virtual consultation with, and I was prescribed a different dose of oestrogen and other natural supplements. That was a game changer for me.

I also set up a group[3] on Facebook a year ago called "Finding me again" which is now going strong and the power of women empowering women has really blown me away.

My overriding recommendation to ladies who are confused or lost about how to deal with their menopause is to seek professional, specialist advice. I believe our bodies need oestrogen and these days you do NOT have to suffer in silence, this is YOUR time. You have worked hard to get here, and you deserve a wonderful happy menopause, not a miserable, painful one. Talk to others, join groups, but above all, see a menopause specialist as I did and start living again; albeit by falling over a lot and making a massive fool of myself as I took up running (which is amazing for clearing the mind and keeping the weight off) and generally seeing the funny side of the brain fog....I regularly turn up to the vet without the dog or take the kids to school and then return home with them still in the car.

For me, laughter has been the best medicine. There is nearly always something funny to be found in life.

[1]*https://menopausalmayhemmothers.home.blog/blogs/*
[2]https://www.menopauseconsultancy.co.uk
[3]*https://www.facebook.com/groups/485385898950382*

Chapter Twelve

Helen Kemp, 48

"When you know better, you do better"

- Maya Angelou -

I would describe the 5 years after my surgical menopause as challenging. Now though, I'm ever so gradually starting to thrive. I can sense my energy levels increasing, I've found my sense of playfulness again, I have a sense of purpose, I want to be alive.

I had a total abdominal hysterectomy including the removal of both ovaries plus fallopian tubes, a TAH-BSO, at the age of 41. I'd had endometriosis, and my ovaries (Otto and Margot) were polycystic. I also had a fruit basket of fibroids, seven in total (they were nameless). Prior to my surgery I waddled around with an abdomen the size of a 5-month pregnancy. I was perpetually uncomfortable and in pain. I just wanted to get the whole lot out and get back to my life.

From seeing the gynae-consultant to the day of surgery was exactly 5 weeks (wow). I was told it could take up to 12 weeks to fully recover from surgery, but that "most women only need around 6-8 weeks". The operation went well although getting on top of the pain proved difficult and I kept being sick.

I'd opted for continuous epidural analgesia (CEA) in addition to a general anaesthetic, on the basis that it would provide the most effective post-operative pain relief. Although I made that decision on the spur of the moment during a pre-op chat with the anaesthetist. As my hospital roommate was up before me on the surgical list, the anaesthetist spoke to her first. Anyone who has ever been in hospital as a patient before will know, a piece of fabric hanging from the ceiling by way of privacy is not an effective sound barrier. I overheard the entire conversation, which included the fact that she was frightened of needles, and on that basis, declined the option of CEA.

That was the point at which my competitive streak kicked in. I have no idea why, and upon reflection it really was an error of judgement, but I decided there and then to go for CEA. I should point out, I wasn't just frightened of needles, I was terrified of needles. I had a full-blown phobia of needles. I routinely fainted whenever I had to have blood taken. Yet there I was readily offering up my spinal canal to a consultant anaesthetist. And all because I'd entered into a game of pain-relief chicken with a fellow patient, who was, I imagine, completely oblivious to my foolish bravado.

Placement of the spinal catheter didn't go as planned, and instead of numbing my surgical site, it numbed only my legs. Periodically throughout the first night after surgery, nurses would arrive at my bedside with 2 small bags containing ice cubes. They would then hold them on various parts of my lower limbs to see if any feeling had returned. It hadn't, although I was in considerable pain around my abdomen.

Eventually the spinal catheter was removed on the basis that at some point I needed to be able to start walking. I can smile now, but at the time, being told by the nurses that I *just* needed to get out of bed and walk around a little to help myself feel better, was rather frustrating, and I felt pretty helpless. I was also more than a little bit concerned that I would never get the feeling back in my legs again. I excel at overthinking ☺ .

To try and get on top of the pain, I was given oral morphine, which just made me sick again. Not ideal. Eventually I was given analgesia in suppository form, which for various reasons proved rather stressful. But, it helped enormously with the pain.

My stay in hospital was a disorientating experience. I suspect mainly due to the lingering effects of the anaesthetic, plus the various pain relief medication. I found it hard to sleep and my face was incredibly itchy, particularly my nose, and I couldn't shift a bad headache. On the second day post-op, I was mobile, and every few hours I would do a lap of the ward, all whilst clutching my abdomen. It was a surreal experience. I felt so fragile and vulnerable.

I was told I would be allowed to leave hospital once my bladder and bowels had both sprung back into life. My bladder duly complied once the catheter was removed but my bowels resolutely refused to perform. After 4 days and unsuccessful encouragement by way of a liquid laxative, I was discharged on the basis that I was likely to be more relaxed at home and nature would eventually take its course. It did, and it wasn't nearly as bad as I'd feared. The one thing you mustn't do is strain. Just relax and breathe. It will be okay.

It's strange the things you take for granted. I needed help opening doors, getting into and out of the car. Every cough or sneeze hurt, and laughing was similarly painful. I missed not being able to stand up straight and have a good stretch. I missed feeling capable.

I left hospital with two instructions: refrain from sex for six weeks and lift nothing heavier than a kettle full of water during the same time period. That was it. In the days and then weeks after surgery, I had no appetite. I was too anxious to eat, not because I thought I would be sick again, I was just too anxious. But I didn't know why. I started to have panic attacks, flashbacks and recurrent nightmares.

I wasn't aware at the time, but the invasive procedures leading up to surgery as well as surgery itself and the acute post-operative period, had triggered issues surrounding unresolved childhood trauma. I'd always thought I'd managed to bury everything sufficiently. It was how I dealt with most things back then, I had a black belt in avoidance.

How many women I wonder have similar experiences? Thankfully there now seems to be a greater awareness around the psychological stress of cervical smear tests and/or pelvic examinations for adult survivors of rape, sexual assault and/or childhood sexual abuse. In December 2020, Dr Karen Treisman MBE published a paper entitled Trauma-Inducing and Trauma-Reducing Health and Medical Experiences[1]. It's well worth a read.

I had multiple trans-vaginal ultrasound scans before and after surgery. I'd lay there watching the nurse putting a condom over the probe. After that, my brain would check out. I'd eventually get off the examination couch shaking. I had no idea where I was.

Pre-existing mental health challenges, plus unresolved trauma, plus menopause equalled an explosion. I've since termed that scenario, the ticking triad timebomb. Gynaecological surgery lit the fuse of my particular timebomb. The net result of which was a breakdown. I resigned from my job and walked away from my career of 20 years.

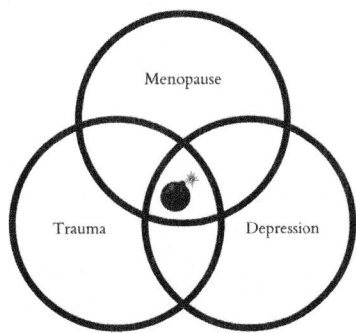

Ticking Triad Timebomb © 2020 Helen Kemp

I wasn't aware that nausea could be part of the experiential milieu of menopause. Ditto anxiety, low confidence, depression, insomnia, brain fog and rage. I only knew to expect hot flushes and/or night sweats, neither of which I had (then). I didn't link the repeated bouts of gingivitis, seborrheic dermatitis, sore knees, elbows and wrists, swollen knuckles, to menopause. I became super anxious about driving, and my spatial awareness seemed to disappear overnight. New symptoms just kept appearing as the months and years ticked by: hair loss, vaginal dryness, itchy skin, dry eyes, restless legs, and on, and on.

A note on vaginal dryness, which as odd as this might sound, wasn't really what I thought it was. Bear with me. Firstly, I'm embarrassed to say I'd mixed up the words vagina and vulva. Secondly, I would get watery, milky discharge, from which I concluded, my tissues were clearly not dry. However, the watery discharge was totally different to what I would have referred to as my normal vaginal discharge, i.e. what I had become accustomed to since puberty. Maybe that should have been my first clue that changes were afoot. Internal examinations became more painful and I picked up one urinary tract infection after another. Then externally, everything seemed to become dry, very dry. Uncomfortably dry. Think sandpaper. I wish the book by Jane Lewis - *Me and My Menopausal Vagina*[2] had been written a decade ago. If you haven't read it, please do. It's an incredibly informative and ground-breaking book.

I also wasn't aware the menopausal transition (irrespective of its nature) could be a particularly vulnerable time in a woman's life with respect to eating disorders[3]. I thought I'd successfully conquered my eating disorder many years ago. However, in the aftermath of my surgery, life felt out of control, and something flicked a switch in my brain. I wasn't eating much as a result of anxiety, plus I was experiencing morning sickness which persisted on and off for a year or so after surgery. As my mental health deteriorated, I started heavily restricting my food intake, and eventually once able, I started to over-exercise.

The first turning point after my hysterectomy was accepting that I had a problem with depression (again), then seeing my GP about it. The narrative is thankfully slowly changing, but we tend to hear very little about the psychological and emotional aspects of menopause.

Antidepressants can get a hard time in the media, but quite honestly, they saved my life, without any doubt. They gave me the first full 8 hours of sleep in over 20 years. I appreciate antidepressants do not work for everyone, but I'm mighty thankful they work for me, and I'm pretty content to accept I may need to take them for the rest of my life. If I had an underactive thyroid, I'd take medication. It just so happens in my case, it's my brain that needs a pharmaceutical intervention.

The second turning point came almost 3 years after the TAH-BSO. I hadn't healed well, and I also had a persistent area of granulation tissue on the vaginal vault which would become uncomfortable and bleed every few months. My life since the hysterectomy had been a protracted ping-pong of appointments back and forth between my GP, gynae-consultant and surgeon.

Initially I wasn't told about the presence of granulation tissue on the vaginal vault. I couldn't understand why I was periodically still bleeding. Quite understandably, I was concerned. My thoughts were, the bleeding is either due to a cancerous growth, a tear in the vault, or due to a regrowth of residual endometriotic lesions. Or worst-case scenario, a combination of all three.

I'd had 4 chemical cauterisations with silver nitrate and my surgeon made it abundantly clear, a 5th round was not an option. Additional surgery was suggested. However, I was adamant I didn't want a fresh round of surgery to try and fix the problem. As a last resort, my surgeon suggested HRT to see if that might improve the situation.

Within a few weeks of starting HRT, the stiffness in my joints disappeared. Over the next six months, my sleep became deeper and more restful, my anxiety became more manageable and my mood stabilised even further. My gums were less sore, my skin didn't itch, and eventually the issue of granulation tissue on the vaginal vault resolved itself and the bleeding stopped.

Energy levels and overall motivation were still a little low, but I'd decided that may well just be the 'new me'. Besides, why was there any need to aim for the 'old me' anyway? And as it turned out, I didn't much like the old me, she wasn't particularly nice, so that was a case of serendipity.

What worked for me, might not work for anyone else. If I've learnt one thing in the years since my hysterectomy, it's that when it comes to menopause, there is no one size fits all, both in terms of symptoms and treatment. Every woman is different.

My approach now is multi-faceted. It involves antidepressants (I take a combination, colloquially known as 'Californian rocket fuel'), HRT in the form of transdermal oestrogen, as well as testosterone. Testosterone is the very latest add-in. I'd tried unsuccessfully for a couple of years to get testosterone via the NHS. In January 2020 I'd spoken to the amazing menopause advocate, Karen Kenning. Karen suggested I make contact with a menopause specialist nurse practitioner in Bristol. Within 7 days of that conversation, I'd had an online consultation and a prescription for Testogel delivered via the post. That's the power and beauty of women supporting women.

Exercise is now a non-negotiable part of my life. I indoor-row 2-3 times a week. I'd seen the awesome Jo Moseley tweeting about her indoor-rowing challenge a few years ago, and that inspired me to give it a go. Weight-bearing exercise is also super important in the fight against osteoporosis, and I run as often as I can. I'm not fast and it's not pretty, but it's exercise and I know I will feel better afterwards.

In mid-2020 I took up Qigong and I find it to be both wonderfully calming and uplifting. It allows me to connect back to my central core spirit. I cannot recommend it enough.

I use cold-water bathing as a means to boost my mood and mitigate hot flushes which started to surface a year or so ago. When the COVID19-pandemic put a halt to my mountain stream bathing, I purchased a large red wheelie-bin. 'Herbert' now sits hidden amongst the trees in my garden. He is full of jolly cold Scottish water, and I hop into him at various times throughout the day, but particularly after exercise when I can find it hard to cool my system.

It's quite amazing that just a few minutes bobbing in Herbert can leave me feeling refreshed, more emotionally buoyant, and I can almost guarantee I will be hot flush free for the remainder of the day. In the future, I am determined to make it to Loch Rannoch, where Dr Melanie Santorini hosts women-only retreats which include the opportunity to swim in the loch.

For the past few years, I've been working with a therapist. Therapy helps me better manage my life as a post-menopausal woman whilst simultaneously navigating cPTSD. Taking responsibility for my wellbeing and my behaviour were crucial, if hard, lessons to learn. I'm now a passionate advocate for talking therapy. I believe seeing a therapist should be just an everyday occurrence, in much the same way we visit a dentist if we have an issue with our teeth. We really need to shift the stigma around therapy.

Any advice or suggestions?

If you have similar surgery to mine, make sure you arrange for a 6-week post-op check-up that involves an examination of the vaginal vault. If something doesn't feel right to you, follow it up and keep following it up. Persistence is key, and I know that's easier said than done, but more often than not we really do know our own body best.

Take someone with you to your appointments. I can find new environments very stressful and overwhelming. Having an appointment buddy is useful not just in terms of moral support, but they can also write down key points that you might forget.

Take a holistic approach to recovery, and to staying recovered. Be open to the possibility of trying a variety of therapies, activities, and medications. Afterall, if you never try, you will never know. If you can, do your own research, and don't always listen to those who shout the loudest (particularly on social media).

Keep checking in with yourself periodically, as you may need to change, add-in, or remove individual components of your wellness toolkit. HRT doses or delivery routes may need to be tweaked, and you may need to shift the emphasis of your workout routines to factor in less high-impact and more load-bearing elements.

Were you prepared for the days and weeks after surgery?

I was in no way prepared for life immediately after my hysterectomy. In light of the comments made by my surgeon, I thought I'd be back up to full speed very quickly. That didn't happen. My recovery was slow and rather protracted. I went back to work eight months after surgery, and I struggled. I could no longer multi-task, I was forgetful, short-tempered, and I couldn't perform some of the more physical aspects of my job, such as shifting 200bar cylinders around the lab. And that really bothered me. I was used to being very capable.

Without doubt I added to my overall stress levels by comparing my recovery to that of other women who'd undergone similar surgery. I felt a failure. I was still trying to be the all-singing, all-dancing version of myself that had existed before surgery. And I couldn't understand where I was going wrong.

I wish I'd been aware...

❖ that a surgical menopause would change me. It changed my entire outlook on life. It forced me to evaluate and recalibrate virtually every aspect of my life, from my career, to my relationships, both with others as well as with myself.

❖ of the impact on my mental and emotional wellbeing. Menopause is so much more than hot flushes and night sweats. Looking back, I'm amazed I didn't notice my mental health deteriorating. I was possibly in denial, but it never occurred to me that I wouldn't simply sail through my menopause. In the days and then weeks after surgery, my mood dropped, my background anxiety levels increased significantly, I was short-tempered and irritable. I didn't want to talk to anyone or see anyone. I just wanted to hide away from the world and go to sleep. I'd navigated depression since my mid-teens and assumed the low mood would eventually pass. It didn't, and I had a return of persistent episodes of suicidal ideation. My life became about getting through each day so that I could go to sleep. In the wee small hours of a bitterly cold December morning in 2017, I'd stood on the bridge over the River Tay in Perth with only one intention. I'd had enough of everything and everyone, including myself.

❖ that my bladder would get itself in a sulk for a week or so after surgery. The sensation of experiencing cramp in my bladder is hard to describe. I needed to spend longer making sure I fully emptied my bladder. I would also need considerably longer to make it to the bathroom. I was used to my brain giving me adequate warning. After surgery though, not only did I take longer to physically walk to the bathroom, but I needed to start making a move in that direction the very second I felt the first twinge. Even then, I still had quite a few accidents.

❖ that it's not uncommon to have pale pink or brown-ish vaginal discharge around 7-10 days post-op as some of the stitches dissolve.

❖ that it will likely take months for the belly swelling to completely reduce. I wasn't back into my pre-op trousers until at least six months after surgery. Even then, my belly would swell up as the day went on and I would often feel a heaviness if I happened to be on my feet for any length of time without a break.

❖ that I would go slap-bang into menopause. I'm not sure why I didn't realise what was going on sooner. However, I know when I'm experiencing a bad episode of depression, I lose my perspective as well as my ability to think logically. Both of those combined with brain fog and insomnia are not optimal conditions for rational thought or meaningful self-reflection.

❖ that having gynaecological surgery could trigger issues around unresolved trauma. I had no idea. In every sense, I had no idea.

What helped in the days and weeks after surgery?

❖ I found holding a pillow tightly against my abdominal incision helpful when coughing or sneezing. I tried to grate cheese about a month after surgery and found it difficult. Who knew to what extent our abdominal and pelvic muscles were involved in such trivial, everyday activities?

❖ Learning how to safely get out of bed by pushing myself up with my arms and then gently rolling over to the side. I need to emphasise the word 'gently'. I was too enthusiastic on one occasion and kept rolling off the side of the bed and onto the floor. Luckily, no harm done but it nonetheless unsettled me.

❖ If you've had an abdominal incision, avoid wearing anything tight around your waist. I wore loose fitting pj's most of the time for a few weeks after surgery. It was a good reminder not just to myself but also those around me that I wasn't firing on all cylinders. Far from it in fact.

❖ Pelvic floor exercises. Thankfully, we're starting to hear more about issues of urinary incontinence, but there still seems considerable shame and embarrassment around fecal incontinence. I lost confidence in my ability to hold onto my stools for the first year after surgery. It's quite a difficult sensation to describe, but my intestines felt 'unstable'. Without doubt pelvic floor exercises have helped enormously. I gradually gained back good control of both my bladder and bowels, although I am still occasionally prone to the odd accident. But, as the saying goes, shit happens.

❖ I signed up to the online community 'HysterSisters'[4] and no matter what time of the day or night, there would be support. No question was too daft and knowing others were experiencing similar issues, provided peace of mind. Other than that, the majority of my information regarding surgical menopause came via Twitter thanks to Dr Hannah Short.

What advice would you offer anyone contemplating a hysterectomy?

Whilst it might be considered routine surgery, it is nonetheless major surgery. Don't compare your recovery to anyone else's. We all heal at different paces. Take as much medical leave as you possibly can to give yourself the best chance of healing and recovering well.

Healing is not necessarily a linear process. Quite often after a few good days, I would be floored by fatigue for a while. Provided the long-term trend is an upwards one, that's all that really matters. Listen to your body. I know that's such a cliché, but it's true.

Get as much information about menopause as you can before surgery. Prepare those around you as well, make sure they know you will likely be physically and emotionally fragile for a while. Irrespective of whether you live alone or with others, its useful to prepare things around the house to make your life easier during the first few weeks. For example, remove any potential trip hazards.

Positives of my menopause experience

My experience of surgical menopause has been incredibly challenging, but it has also been a positive, life-enhancing and life-affirming adventure. I've purposefully used the word 'adventure' there because it would be all too easy to merely focus on the difficult stuff. However, to quote Katherine MacKenett, "mountains do not rise without earthquakes". I wasn't aware of how strong my spirit was, or how resourceful I would become.

My initial struggles have given me a better appreciation of what exactly is important in life. What matters to me above all else is leading a life that best honours my core values. A life that allows me to be my authentic self, to be compassionate, honest and caring.

There are so many positives to surgical menopause, in addition to the very obvious for me, no more heavy, painful and life-disrupting periods. One over-arching bonus is the fact that I now mind less about what other people think of me, and heck that is just so liberating. So, I have a lot to thank my surgical menopause for. I am grateful for how it challenged me to be a kinder, more thoughtful person. For how it laid bare my insecurities. And for how it taught me the value of friendships. I have much to be grateful for.

As a result of my own menopause journey, I became involved with Menopause Café, the Scottish charity. I went along to the world's first ever Menopause Café® in Perth, Scotland and was blown away by the sense of camaraderie and energy in the room. I didn't feel quite so alone in the world, plus I knew I wasn't going mad. My work for Menopause Café now brings me into contact with a vast array of people. I love connecting with folk from all over the world and listening to their experiences and stories.

What helps on a difficult day?

What helps me, first and foremost, is practicing self-compassion. Therapy taught me the importance of compassion, self-care and being kind to myself. I'm a recovering perfectionist and had a tendency to bully and push myself. I now have a much better appreciation of what I need to do to stay emotionally well, and I have a healthier relationship to myself.

I've learnt to change my internal narrative from "that's so pathetic" to "and that's okay". It really helps to be gentle with myself when I'm not feeling great. I also now know when I'm finding the going tough, I need to reach out and connect. As a species, we are not designed to isolate and hide away from the world. And believe me I tried to do just that for too much of my adult life. Find your tribe and stay connected.

My story is not intended to be a tale of woe. I certainly don't see it that way. If I can help prevent others from following in my initial footsteps, then my own struggles will not have been in vain. I appreciate I was fortunate in that I could access a private consultation for HRT. However, I do wonder how much I had spent in the intervening years on a whole variety of supplements designed to either boost my mood, improve my sleep, or stop hair loss. None of which incidentally would have done very much to protect my bone, heart or brain health.

Final thoughts

My plea to those in the healthcare profession; please listen to women, take our concerns seriously, and help us to best help ourselves. Please appreciate that quite often it takes us enormous courage to even walk through your consulting room door. If our concerns are dismissed, it can have a devastating effect on us. It disempowers us, and potentially deters us from seeking further help.

Please don't invalidate our experiences on the basis that "*it's just menopause*". No, it's not "*just menopause*". I don't believe it's an exaggeration to say that I suspect some women will have taken their own lives as a direct result of the impact of menopause. I was almost one of them.

Can we please have better communication and a greater degree of transparency when it comes to sharing the contents of medical notes. I appreciate the NHS is in an incredibly precarious position, however I imagine I would not have needed so many appointments had I been fully briefed about the true nature of my post-surgery complications much sooner.

And very finally, I could not end without bringing up the subject of autism. Receiving my autism diagnosis in 2018 was game-changing. Autism affects every single aspect of my life, and yet there is very little research around autism and female hormonal health overall, and even less about menopause and autism. Yet I hear from women on a regular basis who've received their autism diagnosis at the time of their menopausal transition, invariably as a result of having an acute mental health crisis. I suspect the emotional & physical pressures of menopause tax our executive functioning to breaking point. We can mask no longer. We break.

I am though hopeful that the landscape in relation to the lack of research is gradually shifting, as is evidenced by research published by Moseley[5] et al., 2020. I'm going to quote a paragraph from the authors conclusions. Their observations are tremendously important, and they deserve to be shared as widely as is possible:

"The lack of knowledge around the menopause in autism should, we suggest, be of high concern, particularly given the suggested increase in mental ill-health and suicidal thoughts. Furthermore, the potential exacerbation of social difficulties could thwart communication with health providers at a most vital time".

Alongside my autism, comes alexithymia. I have a problem identifying and describing feelings. I also have sensory processing issues as well as high pain tolerance. The latter may go some way to explain how my endometriosis went undiagnosed for so long, to the point where a doctor told me (simply by looking at my notes) that I couldn't have endometriosis because "no-one presents with undiagnosed endometriosis at the age of 38". Well, I did.

For someone with sensory processing issues, hospitals can quite literally be overwhelming and frightening. Bright lights, loud and unpredictable noises, different fabrics next to the skin, strange smells and unfamiliar foods. And all of those on top of the unavoidable disruption to routine. As an autistic woman, I thrive on sameness, familiar routines and predictability. Any change, even minor, well signposted changes, can be extremely anxiety provoking, and can lead to a complete meltdown.

My surgery was almost postponed due to a large hike in my blood pressure on the day of surgery. It was only because I'd anticipated that might happen and had been monitoring my blood pressure daily in the weeks leading up to surgery, and could produce such records, that the surgical team agreed to proceed.

Being on the autistic spectrum can make daily life extremely challenging and stressful. Nevertheless, with well-judged and timely adjustments, it should be possible to lead a meaningful and enjoyable life. What that life looks like will be different for each and every one of us. However, I am passionate about ensuring that no one is disadvantaged as a result of their neurodiversity.

And now, in early 2021, as the 8th anniversary of my hysterectomy approaches, I am happier and healthier than I have even been before in my life. With the appropriate support, I believe menopause can be a truly liberating time of creativity and spiritual growth. Being kind to ourselves, nurturing ourselves, honouring our bodies and accepting ourselves just as we are, all form the basis for a solid foundation upon which to build this third stage of our lives. Because, we are and always will be, enough.

[1]*Treisman, Karen., 2020 Trauma-Inducing and Trauma-Reducing Health and Medical Experiences: drawing on stories from 390 people and some of the values of trauma-informed practice. http://www.safehandsthinkingminds.co.uk/wp-content/uploads/2020/12/trauma-inducing-or-trauma-reduci.pdf*

[2]Lewis, Jane., 2018 Me & My Menopausal Vagina. PAL Books.
[3]Baker, Jessica H. & Runfola, Cristin D., 2016 Eating disorders in midlife women Maturitas, V85, p112-116.
[4]www.hystersisters.com
[5]Moseley, Rachel L., Druce, Tanya, and Turner-Cobb, Julie M. When my autism broke: A qualitative study spotlighting autistic voices on menopause. Autism 2020 24(6):1423-1437 doi: 10.1177/1362361319901184.

Books which I've found helpful:

❖ Brown, Brené. 2008. I Thought It Was Just Me (but isn't). Making the journey from "what will people think" to "I am enough". Gotham Books.
❖ Gilbert, Paul. 2010. The Compassionate Mind. Constable & Robinson Press.
❖ Henpicked. 2018. Menopause: The Change for The Better. Green Tree.
❖ Joseph, Stephen. 2016. Authentic. How to be yourself and why it matters. Piatkus
❖ Lama, Dalai., Tutu, Desmond and Abrams, Douglas. 2016. The Book of Joy. Lasting happiness in a changing world. Penguin Random House.
❖ Lawson, Wenn. 2015. Older Adults and Autism Spectrum Conditions – An Introduction and Guide. Jessica Kingsley Publishers.
❖ Maté, Gabor. 2019. When the Body Says No. Vermillion, London.
❖ Rothschild, Babette. 2010. Eight Keys to Safe Trauma Recovery. Take charge strategies to empower your healing. W.W. Norton.
❖ Santorini, Melanie. 2019. Majesteria. Spiritual Guidance through the Menopausal Gateway. Balboa Press.
❖ Schwartz, Arielle. 2017. The Complex PTSD Workbook. Althea Books.

Helen works as an independent consultant and advisor. She is passionate about raising awareness of the topics society typically prefers not to speak about, including menopause, childhood sexual abuse, eating disorders, and depression. Helen is an Associate at Equality Counts, and a founding member of the Menopause Inclusion Collective.

Helen describes herself as a gentle, compassionate encourager, and quiet disruptor. Helen is dyslexic and autistic, both of which make her life exciting and perplexing in equal measure. She likes LEGO, Chinook helicopters, and kind, authentic people.

Find Helen on Twitter: @SurMenoNYTM and at www.menopausecollective.org

Section 3

What might help?

1. Exercise

Julie Robinson

Exercise may well be the last thing on your mind after surgery. It was for me when I had a hysterectomy at the age of 36 - and I was a PE teacher. Just trying to stand up straight, get on and off the loo, walk downstairs and make a cup of tea, felt like a marathon. Then there's the shock wave of hormone disruption that comes with surgical menopause that can leave you feeling devoid of energy and enthusiasm. So, when getting out of bed is a trial, why should we even be thinking about exercise?

Firstly, don't think about 'exercise' as you probably equate this with running, squats and the gym. Think of 'movement' as medicine and treat yourself gently at first until you feel ready to consider something more challenging.

The moment you wake from surgery you're encouraged to breathe deeply. Physiotherapists aim to get you moving and out of bed at the earliest possible opportunity even if it's simply squeezing your glutes or pumping your feet to boost circulation. You're most often told not to lift anything heavy for six weeks, not even the kettle, but then have to get into (and out of) a car to get home. It's a bewildering and often scary time.

There's no one size fits all solution as so much depends on your particular situation, medical history, pre-existing fitness and health. This is why you have to rely on your consultant to advise you on when it's safe to resume exercising and if there is anything you must avoid. Generally, it's advised to wait for six weeks after surgery and have been signed off as safe to exercise, although you'll most probably be encouraged to get up and move often and take short walks on level ground. But what then?

Along with advice from a medical professional you now need to be guided by your own body and gradually build up the time and intensity of your chosen exercise. But even before that you need to do your pelvic floor exercises* (unless otherwise advised). Think of your pelvic floor as the foundations to the four walls of a house on which everything above rests and depends. This hammock of muscle runs from your pelvic bone to your tail bone and needs to be exercised every day – not just after surgery, but for life. It may take weeks of pelvic floor exercises before you notice any difference but stick with it, strengthening these muscles will give you the confidence to do other exercises in the future, especially those that are beneficial to your bones which involve some impact.

At first, start off with low impact activities like swimming or brisk walking which are great for heart health. Increase the distance, time or intensity gradually over the next six weeks and make sure you build in rest periods to help you recover. It's better to do two short walks and rest in between than one long walk which leaves you exhausted.

Just a couple of weeks of bed rest leads to a rapid decline in muscle mass. It may be three to six months before you can really start to work-out again but even walking upstairs or getting up and down from you chair repeatedly for one minute every day will help stop your leg muscles from becoming weak.

So, what should you aim to do once you've recovered?

Ideally, we need to do at least 150 minutes of moderate intensity or 75 minutes of high intensity exercise every week. Moderate intensity means doing something that makes you breathe harder, raises your heart rate and makes you feel warm; you should still be able to talk but not sing. High intensity exercise means you can only saw a few words because you're breathing so hard and will be sweating. It's the difference between a light jog and a sprint, or a gentle swim and playing squash.

We also need to do strengthening exercises at least twice a week when you lift, push or pull against a load. This could be using your own body weight, hand-weights, resistance bands or gym machines.

After we hit 30 our bone density starts to decline, then during menopause this accelerates, so doing weight-bearing and bone loading exercise is more important than ever. Any activity that includes some impact such as jumping, skipping or running will benefit your bones. For those who have been diagnosed with osteoporosis, high impact exercises along with extreme forward flexion or twisting should be avoided and replaced with low-impact exercise.

So, in a perfect world we would be swimming, cycling, running, lifting weights, balancing and stretching every week. But what if your joints are aching, you're sleep deprived or you're lacking the motivation, energy or time to get moving? The best way forward is to find something you enjoy, find distraction techniques that help you keep going for longer and remember that every little helps. Bite-size chunks make it far more manageable and give you a sense of achievement – look at what you have done rather than what you feel you should do.

Getting outside for a walk is a great way to get active and doesn't feel like exercise if you're walking and talking with a friend or immersing yourself in a podcast. Consider making the walk a mindful experience and focus on the things you can see, hear, feel, touch and smell along the way. This can help you walk further and begin to look forward to this time when you get some head space and feel great afterwards.

Dancing is a great way to let off steam, lose yourself for a little while and rebalance your mood by releasing those feel-good hormones. Music is one of the best ways to deflect your mind and dancing is a great workout for your heart, muscles, bones and brain. Find somewhere private, turn the music up loud or plug in your headphones, let go of your inhibitions and dance like no one's watching. Another plus is you can burn around 200-400 calories in 30 minutes depending on how energetic your dancing style is.

Make everyday activities part of your 'keep fit' routine. Use the few minutes that it takes to fill the bath to do some squats. Or try balancing on one leg for one minute as the kettle boils (if that's easy then try balancing with your eyes closed). Use the kitchen worksurface to do standing press ups as the pasta is cooking. If you add up all the moments you might not normally use to do some simple activities, it will really start to make a difference, especially if it's a while since you exercised.

As our hormones play a vital role in our mood, exercise can offer a drug free treatment to improve our mental health. This is where group exercise comes into its own; exercising together in a social environment offers an extra dimension. Talking, listening, supporting and laughing with others is a tonic in itself and research shows it's especially beneficial for women going through menopause. Find a group exercise class where the instructor has the knowledge to guide you and the empathy to encourage you to participate with no muscle strains and no feelings of embarrassment.

We can find a hundred excuses not to exercise. Yet if we were offered a drug that could improve almost all of our menopausal symptoms and also reduce our risk of osteoporosis, diabetes, dementia, stroke, heart disease, depression and some cancers, we'd be queueing up to take it. What we choose to do through menopause will hugely impact on our future health, so take some professional advice first and then get moving!

*How to do pelvic floor exercises

First you need to identify the right muscles. The simplest way to do this is to stop urination midstream – if you succeed, you've found your pelvic floor muscles. Only do this once or twice as it can increase your risk of a urinary tract infection (UTI).

There are two types of pelvic floor muscle, slow twitch (which help you maintain control when you have a full bladder and have to wait to get to the loo) and fast twitch (which help prevent leaks when you cough, laugh, sneeze or jump), and you can train them independently.

Slow twitch muscles: need to be recruited smoothly and gently. Tighten the ring of muscles around your back passage as you would if you were preventing yourself from passing wind. Lift the muscles up inside, hold for a second and then relax slowly. Tighten the muscles around your back passage again, now take this feeling through to your front passages. Lift the back and front passages up inside, hold for as many seconds as you can (up to a maximum of ten seconds). Relax the contraction and rest for four seconds then repeat up to 10 times.

Fast twitch muscles: need to be able to react strongly and quickly. Lift up and squeeze the same way you did before but just hold for one second then relax for one second. See how many quick and strong contractions you can do, aim to increase this up to a maximum of ten repetitions, aiming to make the last repetition as strong as the first.

Aim to do your pelvic floor exercises three times a day alternating between slow and fast twitch. Find a trigger that helps you to remember so it becomes a habit, like brushing your teeth. If you're struggling to find the right muscles or find there's no improvement after 12 weeks, then do seek help from your GP. You may benefit from seeing a women's health physiotherapist or being prescribed vaginal pessaries that can improve muscle tone.

For more information on MenoClasses which combine support, discussion and tailored exercise for menopause, see www.menohealth.co.uk or join the MenoSisters Facebook Group www.facebook.com/MenoHealthUK
Find MenoHealth on Twitter: @MenoHealthUK and Julie Tweets at: @FABSJULIE

Julie Robinson had a hysterectomy at the age of 36 and says, "I wish I'd known then what I know now. The decisions and actions we take during this time can affect the rest of our lives. I want to help other women to get the right information and support so they can enjoy healthier, happier lives through menopause and beyond. No one should have to go through menopause feeling alone." Julie founded MenoHealth to make it easier for women to get the support they need and empower them to take control of their menopause.

2. Mindfulness

Becks Armstrong

What is mindfulness?

Mindfulness is a way to become present in the moment. It's a type of meditation that has been researched extensively by psychologists to underscore its efficacy. A lot of time can be spent with the chatter in your mind – thinking about events, people, to-do lists and the future or the past - which means life can feel exhausting or overwhelming. Mindfulness helps you recognise your surroundings and your body without judgement, just awareness.

What does mindfulness do?

One of the main effects of mindfulness is a stress reduction. It can help with lowering the stress hormones in the body. It can help with reducing anxiety, depression and high blood pressure. As a result, it can help you by allowing creative thoughts like planning, problem-solving and controlling your emotions.

What does it not do?

Mindfulness doesn't stop the chatter in your mind, it just slows it down and allows you to get out of a cycle of often unhelpful or busy thoughts. You don't clear your mind to nothing, you simply bring the focus of your thoughts back again and again to a point of focus.

How does it help pre-surgery?

In the lead-up to surgery, many people feel a range of emotions. This can be about what's brought them to the surgery, the procedure itself and how the body will react and how they will feel afterwards. These are all really normal emotions to feel. By sitting in this moment, right now and concentrating on nothing but the feeling of air blowing in and out of your nose, really feeling and noticing the path of air and its effect on the movement of your body, you give your mind and body a break from this stream of thoughts. It can calm the body and allow your mind to put things in perspective. And now you've done a little mindfulness practice!

It can take a little time to get used to the feelings and to slow your mind down, which is why you can use the mindfulness sessions when someone is guiding your thoughts and your breath. You can build up slowly, and many guided mindfulness sessions will be between 5 and 20 minutes.

Suppose you have time to build your practice before your surgery. In that case, it will help you to manage any potential pain and emotional turmoil that can take place. By creating a daily practice of a minimum of 10 minutes twice a day for two weeks, you will start to feel different going into the surgery. It's not a panacea that will stop all anxiety or depression. But a focused practice can help you to reduce the stress and stop the unhelpful spiral of negative thoughts and worries.

Mindfulness in recovery

There may be some pain mixed with emotions after the surgery. If you have had time to build up your mindfulness practice, you can work to acknowledge the feelings in your body without judgement and move your focus to other parts of the body and surroundings. This can help to lower the sensations of pain.

When there are feelings of pain, you can get an increase in cortisol (a stress hormone). This increase in stress hormones can interfere with your anti-inflammatory response and slow your rate of healing. Visualising being aware of your pain, giving it a number on a dial and turning the dial down can sometimes be a helpful way to slowly lower these sensations.

There is a link between mindset and healing. A practice that helps you to lower the stress hormones in the body can help the body to heal.

If you've not had long to practice your mindfulness, then starting now will give you great benefits. They aren't immediate, it does take practice. Finding even 2 minutes to close your eyes, feel where your body is touching the bed, concentrating on all the areas from your head down to your fingers and toes is worthwhile. Two minutes can actually be a long time when you're stressed, so make sure you slowly become aware of where each part of the bed is touching your body. Thinking about how the material feels against your skin or clothing, the difference is between where the material is touching you and where it isn't, can give you a break from your pain and cycling thoughts.

Menopause

One of the main differences for people going through surgical menopause instead of a natural menopause is the sharp change in hormones, which can have a mental and physical effect. Though each person's experience will be different, the fast onset of symptoms can be surprising.

One of the unexpected things that can make a big difference during this period is your mindset. Mindset really matters, which is why mindfulness during this transition phase can really help lower your symptoms and also help to normalise some of the feelings quickly.

There are some things you can do that are simple to help improve your mindset. Writing a daily gratitude journal at night when you go to bed can help you sleep better. The Clarity App has gratitude built into every sleep session because the research is compelling. A positive mindset doesn't mean ignoring reality, it understands that its good anywhere you go looking for it, so start looking for it often!

By taking the time before you go to sleep to think about 5 small specific things that you're grateful for every day, you start to form a shift in your mindset. This does need to be specific though "I'm grateful for my friends" is not specific enough. "I'm grateful that Helen called to check on me today as it made me feel loved" is where you're spending time thinking about the action or event. That's where the magic happens - it stops you from the negative chatter, which then lowers your stress levels and helps you sleep!

If you can keep your 5 (or more if you want) things different and specific, it's usually enough to break the cycle. It's any event or action that happened - it can be enjoying the time to sit and watch leaves falling from trees, family, friends or someone out in the community. Make sure they're different every day, the people may be the same but the event or action needs to change.

By taking the time in your meditation practice to become aware of what you're saying to yourself, you can begin to challenge these thoughts. They are thoughts, not facts, and if they are no longer helping you, you can work to let them go.

Cognitive Behavioural Therapy (CBT) has been proven effective in challenging thoughts and helping you start to let them go. By using some of the CBT techniques in your mindfulness practice, you can start to change the narrative in your mind.

There are 8-week courses called Mindfulness-Based Stress Reduction (MBSR) or Mindfulness-Based Cognitive Therapy (MBCT) that can help you learn to practice mindfulness and how to use it to lower the stress hormones. They don't look specifically at the symptoms of menopause though the practice itself will have a beneficial effect. The MBCT course will help you challenge and improve your mindset specifically.

Wherever you are in your journey, purposefully taking some time out to sit and become aware of your breath, your body and your surroundings is giving yourself some much deserved self-love.

Clarity was made for women by women who know exactly what you're dealing with. You'll find sessions designed specifically to alleviate symptoms of menopause, including: help with falling asleep, stress relief, help to self-soothe during high anxiety and calm a busy mind.

Website: https://clarity.app
Facebook: @ClarityMindfulness
Twitter: @hey_clarity
Instagram: @hey_clarity
iPhone app download: https://apps.apple.com/gb/app/clarity-meditation-for-women/id1375899899
Android app download:
https://play.google.com/store/apps/details?id=com.curiousfu.clarity

Becks Armstrong has dedicated her career to working towards improving the lives of women of all ages and in all situations. Becks founded Clarity to create awareness and support for the issues that uniquely affect women as they get ready for and go through menopause – at whatever age. A trained mindfulness practitioner, doula, and acupuncturist, Becks has a deep understanding of women. She believes with the right access to support, education and information, women can make a real improvement to their lives.

Contact Becks directly at Becks@clarity.app

3. Massage

Elizabeth Bandeen

My name is Elizabeth, and I'm a massage therapist in Glasgow. I am post menopause now, having gone through the main show from 47 to 50 years old. I still get the odd hot flush, which has brought a new friend to the party called nausea, whoop dee doo.

I think that other women in our families are a good indication of how and possibly when we reach menopause, and if we reach it without any other complications or illness accompanying it, then there is so much to be grateful for, but what of others who don't get a choice of how they manage their menopause?

Surgical menopause means that sometimes women can be much, much younger than those of us that it just crept up on, not realising what was happening when we hit the peri-menopause stage. Can surgical menopause be managed? If you are reading this, having gone, or going through surgical menopause then I am excited and also have enormous empathy for you at the same time.

Surgical menopause on one hand means that you are taking a huge step away from the complication that made it necessary, re-occurring oncology, or impossible fibroids, and endometriosis that was not able to be managed, and was crippling you. How amazing to have a medical intervention to get you away from all that, but like many women going through menopause without the surgical interventions being the start point, what next? What support do you have, and what support do you wish you had?

As a massage therapist, and wellness warrior (I was going to write terrier, which I am more akin to but it doesn't sound nearly as glamorous...) the best advice I can ever give to menopausal women is to do your best to remove stress from your life.

In order to make something better, it normally means that you need to subtract something from a situation. If we want to improve mess, we tidy up. When we shower, we wash sweat away. Removing or greatly reducing stress is top of my list when it comes to managing menopause. Also, always have a notebook handy or a diary, to write stuff down that immediately comes to mind, or to plan your day, the night before. Yes, you read that right, plan your day the night before, including what to eat. Don't just leave things to chance and let your day drift along.

So, when you are planning your day, what are you doing for you? What have you got planned that is just for you? I will give you some examples: taking up a hobby. Don't get me started on finger knitting, it's addictive. Is it locking the bathroom door for an hour or so and giving your face a good double cleanse with a hot face cloth and yummy smelling cleansers? Is it booking yourself a massage? Of course, I am going to say that, I am a massage therapist!

Massage is not just great for menopause, it's just great for anyone that really feels like they need it. Why? It's a great distraction, and there is still nothing more alluring than spending a whole hour with someone and all they are focusing on is YOU. Not only is it a fantastic method of stress reduction, but it also helps to clear your mind, helps out with decision making, and makes your central nervous system take a break from all the angst it has been experiencing since your menopausal symptoms started.

An experienced massage therapist will know how to look after you, and I encourage you to go for it. Swedish, hot stones, aromatherapy, reflexology. Knock yourself out. If a client is booking in with me simply for wellbeing and I am not treating an acute injury, booking in between 3 to 4 times a year is fantastic.

With surgical menopause, I thoroughly recommend that when you are fully recovered (post 12 weeks) you do a life inventory. You have changed and for the better. You have had surgery to get you further away from the complications that were consuming you and your health before, but now you have new things to deal with, and trying to knacker yourself out with high intensity exercise and starving yourself because you ate a whole pack of biscuits is not the way forward. Be kind to yourself, give yourself time and space.

Here is my 5-minute win list:

- Go through your work/personal/home areas of life to figure out how to remove stress. If walking into your house to be confronted by a pile of shoes at the door is naffing you off, let's change it!
- Plan your meals and don't ever let yourself go hungry because that's when you'll reach for stuff that can possibly trigger a hot flush and other symptoms. Eat as well as you can. Boiled eggs for breakfast for the win. If you eat more protein, your body will crave less sugar.
- Pilates/yoga/cycling for the win.

- Have a great bedtime routine, that includes not having your phone on charge next to your bed. Make sure that your bedroom doesn't look like the Death Star when you turn the lights off.

So, there you have it. A massage therapists view on how to look after yourself post-surgery. What an amazingly brave decision you have made, or maybe you didn't have a choice, to preserve your life, so that you are still here for your family, friends, and the rest of us who have still yet to meet you.

I grieve for the loss of your ovaries. I know it sounds odd. I did actually grieve for mine when the 'shop shut' as I said to my Mum. I am however excited for you. You are still here, and whatever you have been through, you are in a valuable position to help others with your wisdom if you choose.

Website: www.elizabethbandeen.co.uk
Elizabeth tweets at: @bestevermassage

4. Qigong

Clare Lawrence-Simms

"As the breath settles, the body settles, and as the body settles, the mind settles."

I came to Qigong in my early 40s during an episode of depression and fell in love with it from the first breath. The gentle, forgiving movements were easy to do and learn, soothing my anxiety and bringing me a peace like nothing else I had ever experienced. I attended a weekly class, and it became a daily practice for me; after about 3 years I trained to lead sessions and loved that this allowed me to connect to supportive, like-minded people.

Qigong means "energy work" and this healing art is completely holistic, working with the body, mind, emotions, spirit and energy to give the practitioner exactly what they need when they need it. Also known as moving meditation, Qigong perfectly complemented and embodied the mindfulness that was already helping me to manage my unruly mind. The Shibashi Qigong set that I practise is designed to bring perfect balance on all levels. Through it I have learnt better posture and how to regulate my emotions, which have a tendency towards both extreme highs and extreme lows.

In Qigong we help to settle the mind by focusing on the breath and the body. Relaxing the body allows energy, blood and life-giving oxygen to circulate and nourish every cell as well as carrying away and releasing what the body doesn't need. The same process happens for the emotions. As the owner of a busy brain, I find it very rare that I have no thoughts, but the thoughts that flow during Qigong do so gently and tend to be of a high quality.

The moves are deceptively powerful; initially most people are seeking relaxation and the focus is on simply enjoying the experience. However, in a similar way to yoga and Pilates, as one progresses, the internal and core muscles are developed rather than the obvious outer muscles that tend to be developed in "Western" forms of exercise.

Qigong builds strength from the inside out, both in terms of physicality and mentality. Through Qigong I have learnt to be grounded in my own space and to find my place in the world. My sense of self-worth has grown, and I can recognise how I fit into the natural world as well as the world of humanity. It has helped me to become more self-aware and also to understand and appreciate others more. Qigong is not about pushing, straining and "going for the burn", it is about gently expanding our capacity over time. Wherever we are on a particular day is enough and for me this idea was liberating.

I have never had a comfortable relationship with my body and my mind has always driven me with ridiculous expectations and pressure. I have always been clumsy and awkward physically and for a lot of my life hated myself on all levels.

Qigong has freed me from a lot of this mental tyranny. Firstly, it connected me to my body and taught me to listen and understand its needs and messages. I was able to feel graceful and beautiful as I moved; subsequently it has enabled me to accept and finally love my body and the person that I am. It has helped me to develop confidence and when the menopause threw digestive difficulties, insomnia and severe anxiety at me it gave me a lifeline. No matter how I am feeling, Qigong always makes me feel better.

As Debbie Gannon[1] (to whom I am eternally grateful) states, "Qigong is a way of life". It opens up our bodies, minds and spirits, encouraging healing on all levels. Qigong has brought vibrancy and flow into my life. I love the beautiful names of certain moves and the imagery, which gives free rein to my creativity, helping me to make sense of being human.

Learning to lead Qigong sessions has assisted me in finding my place professionally as I have struggled throughout my life with anxiety in the workplace. It has given me a voice through giving presentations and talks about it.

Each time I practise Qigong I learn more about this art, myself, the world and others. For me it is a celebration of the whole of life, yin and yang, "good" and "bad", masculinity and femininity. It has enabled me to nurture my masculine side and empower my feminine side.

Qigong is designed to be practised outside in nature. I especially love to be by the sea when doing it and have experienced some profoundly blissful moments, unlike anything offered by our modern lifestyle. Someone I worked with, a former drug addict, likened this sense of bliss to the high she would get from cocaine.

The benefits of Qigong for me have been far reaching. It has taught me self-responsibility since it is up to the individual to know their own limits and the only rule is that nothing should hurt on any level. Each person needs to be guided by the session leader and find their own way of performing the set. This was difficult for me, as it is for many women who are used to doing things "perfectly" and judging themselves by someone else's standards. This art has helped me to have the courage to do what is right for me.

Initially I found it quite difficult to perform the moves with the slowness and "stillness" of my teacher. However, as I have progressed, I have grown to love the unhurried nature of the art and this has spread into my everyday life. My patience has increased, and I am much more at ease with myself, others and life in general. The aim is to be able to "be" the moves, rather than "do" them and the energetic benefits mean that they are suitable to be adapted to the requirements of any state of health.

The moves can be performed standing, seated, lying down or mentally and simply being present during a Qigong session enjoying watching others and absorbing the energy can be very powerful. Qigong has helped me to recognise the true wonder of simply being alive, as me, in this world, as it is. To me it is magic, pure and simple and available to us all.

Anyone who has experienced surgery needs to follow the advice of their medical consultant regarding their own limits. According to Debbie Gannon[1] "an experienced practitioner of Qigong would be practising Qigong before, during and after recovery as an aid to healing".

[1] *Debbie Gannon, Shibashi Training Academy www.shibashitraining.co.uk*

Website: www.claritywithclare.co.uk
Clare tweets as: @oadbyfsf

5. Wellbeing

Heidi Dodson

It's important to make wellbeing a priority during menopause. Keeping our physical health and emotional wellbeing front and centre will never be more important. We need to ask ourselves, what's working for us, and what isn't. Surgical menopause can be quite brutal and taking the time to allow our bodies to heal and recover is vital. Knowing when to ease up and be kind to ourselves can be challenging, especially when we're used to being all-things to all-people.

Equally important is ensuring that everyone takes the time to look out for each other. Menopause can leave women feeling isolated and alone. Sometimes just checking-in with someone, maybe by sending a text message can make all the difference. Having access to professional help that focuses solely on your wellbeing is another really powerful way to make sure this stage of your life is as happy, stress-free and productive as you want it to be.

I've listed below my top ten tips for looking after yourself. I know most of them are just plain, old-fashioned common sense, and yet how many of us truly take pleasure in looking after ourselves. None of the below cost very much, and perhaps that's the beauty of them. It might be that you can initially only manage two on the list, but that's a great place to start!

Here are my top ten tips for looking after yourself during menopause.

1. Sleep
    Aim for 8 hours, no social media or screen time 2 hours before bedtime.

2. Exercise
    Find something you love, is there something you loved doing as a child?
    Ride a bicycle, run, go for a walk – all are free!

3. Fun
   Watch a comedy, laugh out loud, connect with friends who make you laugh.

4. Regular breaks
   Meditation Apps, five-minute breaks where you do absolutely nothing, take a power nap...I particularly love this one ☺ .

5. Drinks
   Limit alcohol and coffee. Increase water, fresh juices and smoothies.

6. Surround yourself with the right people
   Talk to people you can trust and have positive, motivating conversations.

7. Mental health
   Talk to someone about your fears or write them down to get them out of your head. Speak to a professional, it's good to talk and they love listening.

8. Work
   What do you love about your job? Find the positives and focus on them.

9. Meals
   Plan your meals for the week, include at least 5 portions fruit & vegetables.

10. Reward yourself
   Treat yourself if you achieve a goal.

To learn more about health and wellbeing in menopause, simply contact me and we'll take it from there.

Website: www.heididodson.com
Facebook: @heididodsoncoaching
Twitter: @wellness_heidi
Instagram: @heididodson2020
LinkedIn - https://www.linkedin.com/in/heidi-dodson-a83213130/

Heidi Dodson is a Counsellor, Life Coach, Relationship Therapist and Fitness Instructor.

6. Yoga

Geraldine Norris

"Take advantage of the clarity of vision that is the gift of menopause and use that gift to let the second half of your life truly be your own."

- Dr Christiane Northrup -

I am 54 years young and have been practicing yoga for four decades and teaching for almost 30 years. I have adapted my own yoga practice during chronic illness, grief, pregnancy, postpartum, as a busy working mother and now at peri-menopause to suit my needs and in doing so the needs of others.

My greatest resource are my students as I always learn so much from them, especially when they present with various medical conditions, injuries, life-events. In addition, my own yoga practice has changed dramatically over the years through my own life's journey.

What is Hatha Yoga?

The word 'Yoga' comes from the Sanskrit word 'yuj' to 'yoke', 'unite' – a union of mind, breath and body with Universal Energy. Hatha Yoga is often described as the physical path of yoga and has become popular here in the West.

The Sanskrit word 'Hatha' literally means 'force' and consists of two letters: Ha meaning 'Sun' which never sets and represents our soul (Atman) and 'Tha' meaning 'Moon', or reflected light of the sun, symbolising consciousness, the reflected light of the soul.

Why Yoga for 'Hot' Women?

Just over a year ago I began teaching Yoga for 'Hot' Women classes. 'Hot' Women is a term I use referring to peri-menopausal and menopausal symptoms in women, not necessarily hot flushes and night sweats as not all women suffer with those symptoms.

I wanted to tailor a short course of Hatha Yoga practice specifically tailored to support, nourish and empower women through some of the many symptoms encountered at peri-menopause, menopause and beyond.

Interestingly the menopause is often referred to as 'the change' and I believe Hatha Yoga is key to helping us, not just on a physical level, but to navigate through this period of transition to unite with our true-self, and fulfil our destiny, our 'calling', soul's purpose so to speak. It is indeed a time of change, transformation, a metamorphosis as major shifts occur in our endocrine system, often a journey of self-discovery, leading to life-changing events. A time to slow-down, take stock and reflect on who we truly are and what we want from life.

I love to investigate, explore, watch, listen, read, learn and have gleaned so much knowledge, tried and tested various methods of yoga practice, plus other coping strategies that help me at this stage in my life. I am keen to share my knowledge and experience, as a yoga teacher, yoga practitioner, homoeopath and a woman, confident it will help to empower, nourish and support other women.

I have become increasingly aware of menopausal symptoms and the impact they have on so many women who are suffering, often in silence, wondering what the hell is happening to them! This seems particularly true in the case of surgical menopause, often resulting in hormonal chaos and a fast-track menopause.

The majority of women in my classes have benefited from a hysterectomy after years of suffering with various health issues: menstrual symptoms, painful endometriosis, fibroids, uterine cancer, etc. Although they often encounter a host of other symptoms post-surgery, possibly not experienced before, such as: depression, brain-fog, hot flushes, aching joints, insomnia, osteopenia, osteoporosis, vaginal atrophy, to name but a few.

Yoga practice can help reduce some of the more undesirable effects of hormonal changes by helping to restore balance and harmony to every system of the body and mind. Yoga is far more than 'physical postures'. However, Instagram is full of wonderfully toned, younger yoga practitioners in various, often quite challenging yoga poses. I wish I had a £1 for every time a person has said to me "I'd love to do yoga but I'm just not flexible enough". I take pleasure in telling them that yoga is not about tying ourselves in knots but untying them.

What to expect in Yoga for 'Hot' Women classes?

I teach a variety of yoga techniques to help cope with some of the many symptoms that can occur around menopause e.g., irregular and/or heavy periods, hot flushes, sweats, pelvic-floor issues, pains in the joints, mood swings, sleeplessness, anxiety, depression, panic-attacks, 'brain-fog', headaches, palpitations, bone health, fatigue, loss of libido, etc.

We also explore the importance of nutrition, exercise, relaxation, mindfulness, self-care and a variety of treatment options. The group share their experiences and coping strategies, so we learn from each other which is often very reassuring and supportive. We also laugh, be sad, confused, hot, cold, anxious, depressed sometimes. I teach my students to recognise, acknowledge and accept these emotions as part of the process as we journey through life. There is light at the end of the tunnel, even if you sometimes feel lost in the dark.

How soon after a hysterectomy can I practice yoga?

A general guideline is to wait 6/8 weeks before commencing physical activity such as Hatha Yoga, however, this depends on individual circumstances, the type of surgery, level of fitness before surgery, individual recovery and healing process.

Many of the yoga postures will be contraindicated initially, to safeguard the wound(s), but an experienced yoga teacher will offer alternative postures, and/or modifications, as there is a risk of injury after hysterectomy and other surgical procedures. Post-surgery, if you are lucky, you will receive physiotherapy which will help you on your road to recovery. Always seek advice and guidance before starting yoga or any other physical activity. Rest really is best to heal.

A Yoga Student Health Questionnaire should preferably be completed before attending yoga classes/courses. Where there are medical conditions, injury, recent surgery or treatment programmes e.g., IVF, the instructor should always advise the student to check with their medical professional or therapist before commencing yoga sessions.

What yoga techniques do I use and teach?

MINDFULNESS

Awareness of our body, mind, breath, all our senses, surroundings, encounters with others and how we interact. Yoga teaches us to be in the moment and experience it fully, with all our senses, breathing, living it with total awareness. "Relaxation techniques and a mindful attitude can reduce symptoms of menopause"[1].

This technique can be particularly useful in helping to ease anxiety, brain-fog, depression, hot flushes, night sweats, chills, itching, etc., by noticing any possible triggers. Practicing mindfulness can be quite revolutionary and life-changing for the better. An example may be that caffeine or alcohol, or spicy food intake may precede a hot flush. By becoming mindfully aware, you can control the intake of these substances and take note of any subsequent changes.

On a practical level I use mindfulness to help combat the absentmindedness I sometimes experience during peri-menopause. When I leave the house it's like a game of 'head, shoulders, knees and toes', however for me it's 'glasses, bag, keys and phone'! I teach mindfulness and many of my students use a variety of 'Apps' to support their practice.

MEDITATION

Honestly if I can meditate anyone can as I've one of the busiest brains I know! I am passionate about many things and meditation is one of them. If you are 50+ I am sure you will remember the Mary Hopkins song "I'd like to teach the world to sing, in perfect harmony?" Well, I'd like to teach the world to meditate in perfect harmony!

Meditation doesn't have to be practiced sitting, in fact I pride myself on making mediation accessible to the masses – washing the dishes, walking, running, dancing, singing, painting, knitting, crocheting, embroidering, building, creating, etc. Our minds have the magical ability to switch to a different frequency for restoration and to reboot, where the parasympathetic nervous system becomes engaged, resulting in a wonderful feeling of peace, tranquillity, calmness and relaxation.

How often have you or someone you know been watching TV, staring out of the window on a car/bus/train journey, gazing at a real fire and have zoned out completely? When questioned, you/they are unable to recall what they were looking at as their mind had wandered from what was in front of them. That is meditation!

According to www.wellbalancedwomen.com "Scientific studies show that a practice of silence, like meditation, can bring relief from common menopause symptoms".

PRANAYAMA (SPECIFIC BREATH CONTROL EXERCISES)

Breath control is paramount to our physical and mental wellbeing. The breath provides instant and reliable feedback to help navigate what is happening within and without. Many of the specific yoga breathing exercises can be used to help relax the body, energise it, cool it down, warm it up, etc. This can be particularly useful in easing hot flushes, panic attacks, anxiety, night sweats, insomnia, or brain-fog. The good thing is gentle breathing exercises can be used almost immediately post-surgery to help oxygenate the system, speed up recovery, enhance our feel-good factor, support mindfulness and meditation practices.

MUDRA (SEAL, MARK, GESTURE)

The most common Mudras are known as 'Hasta' (hand) Mudras, but others involve other parts of the body. These symbolic gestures are a physical expression which has a psychic resonance. Many students benefit from the use of mudras to help ease insomnia, restlessness, anxiety, fatigue and tone the pelvic floor. <u>Some mudras are quite physical and may be contraindicated initially after a surgical menopause.</u>

BANDHA (LOCK)

These are muscular contractions that help seal and move the body's natural energy flow. They can be very toning for the pelvic floor and abdomen, however, not advisable in the early stages of recovery after abdominal surgery. It is always best to practice under the supervision of an experienced yoga teacher who can advise on contraindications and offer modifications.

ASANA (POSTURES)

The yogis tell us that we are as young as our spine is flexible. In a well-balanced Hatha Yoga session you will enjoy a physical warm-up to each series of postures that should include forward/back/side bending, twisting and a balance. Yoga asana not only stretches and relaxes us physically but combined with deep breathing and conscious awareness, they work on every system of the body, mind and breath.

Specific postures will have specific benefits for certain parts of the body. The benefits are many and you should feel more balanced, confident and relaxed after a physical yoga practice.

In an article published in June 2003 edition of www.yogaandhealthmag.co.uk titled "Yoga Turns Back the Clock" by Glenda Twining, benefits listed by The International Association of Yoga Therapists included: increased cardiovascular efficiency, decreased blood pressure, improved posture, increased immunity, decreased hostility and depression, improved balance, improved memory and concentration.

RELAXATION

Our bodies are often like a coiled spring, full of tension, and few know how to truly let go of that tension and relax. Yoga teaches you how, and this will become an integral part of your self-care.

I hope I have whetted your appetite for Yoga, and I wish you a magical life's journey. If you want to discover more, I recommend this website: *www.biharyoga.net*

[1]www.mindfulnessuk.com

Website: www.aurayoga.co.uk
Facebook: @aurayogauk
Geraldine tweets as: @Geraldi10274783

Geraldine Norris is a qualified Yoga instructor with over 30 years of teaching experience who describes Yoga as a 'Science for Life' that has and continues to sustain her. She is passionate about making Yoga accessible for all regardless of background, health, fitness levels, age and experience. Geraldine offers 'Introduction to Meditation' courses and hosts a well-established Yoga Meditation Group via Zoom.

7. Coaching

Laura Shuckburgh

When we start the journey into menopause it can be a massive shock to our systems. Especially when brought on suddenly or prematurely. The changes that our diminished hormones have on our bodies and our minds can be overwhelming.

"I think when you approach mid-life, it's easy to feel half a person compared to your younger dynamic self and not see the qualities that age and experience can bring."

Every woman's journey is totally unique. However, there are symptoms that many women typically experience during menopause including anxiety, depression, loss of confidence, or feeling like half of them is missing. "I just don't feel like myself anymore" is a common theme, along with the physical symptoms. This potent cocktail can be inconvenient for some and debilitating for others.

And it is true, we have lost part of ourselves, our hormones, and this brings up so much for us as women. There can be a kind of mourning for our bodies heading away from our childbearing days and into a new phase. While this is something to be celebrated and embraced, for many women it feels more like a time for grieving. Unless we acknowledge and allow these feelings to be felt, we can easily become very unhappy and 'out of sorts'.

This is where coaching can be beneficial. A coaching session is a completely safe space, a confidential container where women are listened to deeply, can be open and talk frankly about how they are feeling in a non-judgmental place. Coaching focuses on the future not the past. The emphasis is on the present and what is possible going forward. It's about finding solutions for what is not serving or working anymore. It is a place to grow, evolve and create.

"I left feeling at peace with myself and with a strong sense of direction in terms of what I needed to do for me"

Self-doubt can sabotage our dreams and goals. We can be our own worst enemy at times. Noticing our negative self-talk and creating kindness and self-care regimes can be extremely helpful. For many women, this is the first time they've had time and space to give these ideas any thought and to focus some much-needed energy on themselves. Coaching can help make sense of where to go next in this journey of life. It can help us to live a life that is congruent with our values and therefore one that makes us truly happy. In that sense, time spent working with a life-coach could be thought of as "a mental spa day".

Menopause can bring up many questions within us about life purpose and fulfillment. This can lead to confusion and internal turmoil. For most women, thinking about what they want as opposed to trying to please and care for all those around them is something new and potentially uncomfortable. Coaching can be a way to explore this without feeling guilty.

Website: www.marvellousmidlife.co.uk
Facebook: https://www.facebook.com/marvellousmidlife
Twitter: @marvelousmidlif
Instagram: @marvellousmidlife
Linkedin: www.linkedin.com/in/lshuckburgh/

Laura Shuckburgh is a life and transformation coach. She runs a coaching practice under the brand name of Marvellous Midlife. Laura works with women one-to-one online, as well as with organisations where she delivers menopause awareness sessions and manager training workshops.

8. Arvigo® Techniques of Mayan Abdominal Therapy (ATMAT)

Tara Ghosh

I'm sure you're wondering, what on earth is Arvigo® therapy? ATMAT is a non-invasive, external massage technique that is said to improve blood flow and circulation to all the organs in our abdomen. Around the world, cultures have used abdominal massage since time began and ATMAT has its roots in Mayan culture from Central America. It was created by Dr Rosita Arvigo who combined her training as a naprapathic doctor, with the teachings of many traditional healers including Don Elijio Panti, a Mayan Healer. Don Elijio Panti worked all his life healing with hands on techniques and herbal remedies.

In the aftermath of a surgical menopause, women can experience a disconnect between themselves their bodies and their femininity. It's worth remembering that women will, in an energy sense, always have their "womb space". Spending time working with an abdominal massage therapist can help women to reconnect back to their central core energy. When helping clients to prepare for menopause, I typically recommend a multi-pronged approach encompassing nutrition, looking after gut health and the digestive system, and importantly, stress management.

A healthy diet really is the bedrock of your wellbeing and here are my 3 simple tips:

1. Aim to eat protein and healthy fats with every meal. Sources of so-called "healthy fats" include nuts, seeds, olives, avocados, eggs and cold-water fish like salmon and sardines.

2. We ideally want each and every meal to be 50% vegetables. Yep, you read that right, 50%! This is the gold standard I ask clients to reach for, but obviously not every day will be like that, so be kind to yourself and focus on adding veggies whenever and wherever you can. What vegetables should you be eating? Try to eat the whole rainbow of vegetable colours as this promotes a good microbiome, and during

menopause you especially want to eat lots of green leafy vegetables, and to have nutrient dense, fibre-rich foods.

3. The last thing to remember is that we need to eat slowly and with a smile on our face. Believe me, this simple change to our eating habits is really important. We ideally should chew each mouthful 15-20 times, but I like to make it super easy for people, and say let's try to chew at least 10 times per mouthful. A trick to make this doable is to put down your cutlery between each bite and don't pick them up again until you have chewed 10 times and swallowed that mouthful. Why is eating slowly important? Digestion is a team effort starting with chewing which cues the rest of your digestive system to be ready for the food. When we eat more slowly, we can reduce what we eat by up to a third as the hormone, leptin, which tells us we're full, has time to kick in. Now that's reason alone to eat slower.

The period of recovery following surgery can often be a timely opportunity to reflect on what elements within our lives are serving us well. This is obviously a huge topic, but I want to first acknowledge that there is a societal expectation that we must always be "on" and available. However, we underestimate modern life's unrelenting emotional, psychological and physical stress and the effect it has on our overall health. Taking time to audit and then address our stress levels can play an important role in helping us all stay happier and healthier throughout our post-menopausal years.

That's why it's important to have good self-care so we can limit the impact of what modern life bombards us with. We must prioritise our sleep, as well as making sure self-care, in whatever form, is part of our daily routine. Just like we brush our teeth twice a day to make sure we have healthy teeth and gums, and we would never skip that, we need to proactively do self-care every day to ensure we are well mentally and physically as we move through menopause.

Self-care ideas that you can try include meditation and visualisation, breathing techniques, time in nature and exercise, and of course massage therapy! Try a few and see which you enjoy, as the habits that are fun are the ones we can stick to. I wish you all the very best on your health journey.

As with most therapies, there are contraindications and I always recommend clients seek clearance first from their GP before receiving ATMAT.

Website: https://taraghosh.com
Facebook: @TaraGhoshArvigo
*Instagram: @_taraghosh_*

Tara Ghosh is an Arvigo® Therapist and holistic health consultant passionate about empowering women to feel strong whatever season of their life they are in. Tara runs online workshops sharing ways to boost your immunity, improve your libido and balance your moods.

9. Navigating yourself back into the workplace

Sarah Williams

I went back to work too soon. Out of sheer delight at being released from the monthly chaos of PMDD and feeling a sense of anticipation for my new life after surgery, I said 'yes' to too many opportunities too soon, and not enough yes's to quiet recovery time.

With the menopause conversation also taking off in the public sphere, I was inundated with requests for training sessions on top of my usual freelancing work. This felt like a positive start to my new chapter and I embraced every request with a yes, yes, yes!

I was not however, heeding my own wellbeing guidance, after all, they do say a plumber's tap is always dripping! Rather than taking time to get to know and understand the new limits of my post-surgical menopause brain and body, I was within a year, flat out, overwhelmed, exhausted, and slipping into a fast route to 'Burnoutsville'.

My brain and body refused to cooperate indefinitely though, and in the summer of 2020, after 18 months of ignoring all the signs, I had to concede to needing time-out, proper staying-in-bed rest. Getting back to me and getting back to work has taken an applied approach to nutrition, lifestyle and taking my own advice in having a more mindful approach in accepting this new life phase.

My journey to this time out was not solely caused by my surgery, but the operation and how I managed my recovery *was* a huge factor. How I have addressed this time is maybe a tale for another chapter in another book sometime, but burnout, chronic fatigue syndrome and stress-management have all gone from being conditions I've never considered before to terms in daily use now.

So, if you feel exhausted, like too tired to move a limb, like your limbs are sunk deep and heavy like stone into your mattress, or your legs feel like wading through a bog of treacle, or every time you look at your laptop you burst into tears, then you are likely exhausted and need to take action to rest and recover, not keep working!

I've almost had to dial back 18 months and revisit my recovery from surgery and am now taking the slower approach I should have taken then! I just did too much too soon. It is important to rest as much as you are able to, when you need to, and that includes managing your approach to work and being open to reaching out for help when you need it.

Most of us will have to return to work after surgery though, whatever your personal circumstances dictate, try to avoid going back to work too soon if you don't feel ready. Take time to understand the implications for your mind and body in returning to work, consider how your role might be impacted and what support you might need to be able to perform at your best.

It's important to know though, that you do have support of sorts on your return. Where menopause related symptoms have a 'substantial' and 'long-term' negative impact on your ability to do normal daily activities, this may, in some circumstances, give rise to protection under the Equality Act 2010. There have already been several successful claims of discrimination against the protected characteristics of Age, Disability and Sex. A quick internet search will give you more information into the details of these cases, and employers do well to be forward thinking and informed.

On returning to work, plan ahead for how you will manage any troublesome symptoms as once you are back in the workplace this is not always easy, especially if you're feeling overwhelmed, in low mood, or anxious about how your menopause status is being perceived in your workplace. It helps for you to have your plan in place *before* you return.

Although you're under no obligation to tell anyone about your menopause status, it might be helpful for you to talk to your Line Manager about any challenges you're having. After all, if they aren't aware you need support, they will be unable to help you.

Some tips for approaching this meeting:

Ask for a meeting to talk about menopause. If you want the best outcome for you, then having a line manager that is aware of the basics of menopause is helpful. They don't need to know your intimate issues, or be able to advise you on treatments, but a basic understanding of how symptoms can affect workplace performance is a good place to start for your conversation.

If your employer isn't yet menopause friendly, when you request your meeting, you could include a link to a reputable organisation using evidence-based research, so your manager has time to find out about menopause ahead of you getting together. The British Menopause Society[1] has guidance about menopause in the workplace as does The Chartered Institute of Personnel Development[2] (CIPD), or, if your workplace works alongside support from a Union, they may have a menopause toolkit in place.

Plan what you want to say, think about how the conversation might go, *both ways*, have a plan of what you will do if it doesn't go as you expect it to too. Think about the situations at work that are causing you difficulty and what the potential solutions might be. If you take a solution to your line manager rather than a 'problem' you are more likely to reach an outcome that is favourable to you.

Speak with your line manager about your symptoms, how you are feeling and how your work is being affected. You could ask for a reasonable adjustment passport to manage and record your agreed temporary adjustments. This will minimise repeated stress on you by having to repeatedly disclose your situation, remind people about your agreements and your passport can go with you to a new role or line manager.

If the thought of disclosing your menopause is overwhelming, consider taking a trusted work colleague, or 'Menopause Champion' to the meeting with you, let your line manager know ahead of time that you will have company. You can also speak to someone in HR or Occupational Health if this is preferable and available to you. Just think what a relief it will be to have talked about how you are feeling and to have started the conversation about any reasonable adjustments you need.

Your workplace toolkit:

Taking time to plan and prepare your workplace toolkit can make all the difference to how you experience your workday. Here are a few helpful workplace tips that will empower you to be more able to thrive at work.

Your toolkit might include those reasonable adjustments such as a desk fan, and it might also include your own personal wellbeing items like an aromatherapy roller, or a mindfulness App, wet-wipes, headphones, an herbal tea, a healthy snack to lift your mood and energy, and other items that help you to feel calm and supported at work and able to freshen up at work.

Take some time to list the symptoms you are having difficulty with and the reasonable adjustments that might help you:

- ❖ A desk fan to help through hot flushes
- ❖ Is there a desk by a window that would suit you better?
- ❖ The ability to work in a quiet space if you're experiencing headaches or overwhelm from noise levels

❖ Is there a darkened room for you to take time out in if you have migraines, do they have the facility to install a dimmer switch in your office?
❖ Can you have a locker or a facility to store a change of clothes in case of hot flushes and/or heavy bleeding/flooding leaving you needing a change of clothes?
❖ Might you need an extra break to take a quick mindful walk to help lift your mood?

Make a plan for what you will do in case of overwhelm, including thinking about who will be your menopause buddy at work? Who is best placed and trusted by you to help you navigate those tricky days at work, whether working at home or from the office? If there's no one to hand who can you call or text for support? So, make a note of:

❖ Who will you go to for help?
❖ What technique will you use to help you feel better? Mindfulness? Paced breathing? A quick walk?
❖ Where will you go to do this? Is there a designated 'take 10' room in your workplace? Can you have a planned walking route that you know will help you to unwind?

To discover what support is available to you at work, get to know your workplace 'Menopause Champion'. If there isn't one, is this something you would consider doing?

As awareness of the issues surrounding managing menopause at work rises, more claims will be made. It's of benefit to your employer to understand how they can best support employees going through the menopause. This can prevent them from unwittingly engaging in discriminatory practices.

Press for change in your workplace to ensure conversations about menopause and surgical menopause are taking place. Ask for awareness workshops, training for leaders and ask for a Menopause Café[3] at Work. They're great places to chat safely about menopause. If there are no plans for this in your workplace, could it be you that establishes the Café?

During my journey through peri-menopause, PMDD and post-surgery, I started freelancing in the field of equality, diversity and inclusion as an Independent Advisor and Trainer. As a result of my own experiences, the focus of my work has shifted substantially. I've now placed a greater emphasis on empowering and enabling women and workplaces to better manage menopause at work. I achieve this primarily by delivering awareness and training workshops for whole staff teams and managers in the public sector, 3rd sector, and with local government organisations across Wales.

I feel privileged to have been able to turn a challenging personal experience into a force for good. I'm continually humbled by the incredible women I meet with the most amazing stories of how they are attempting to juggle health, home and work life through this phase. I'm also inspired by the men I have met in these organisations who are so keen to understand menopause and champion the cause. I feel hopeful that change is coming!

In all of my work I try to encourage conversations around difficult and taboo topics by creating a safe and non-judgmental space. This is particularly relevant when facilitating discussions on equality, diversity, inclusion, and menopause. I also like to enjoy a bit of laughter and my courses are professional but there will always be a little bit of fun! I was pleased to have featured on BBC Wales, S4C and ITV Wales, where I spoke about menopause and PMDD.

[1]https://thebms.org.uk/publications/tools-for-clinicians/
[2]https://www.cipd.co.uk/knowledge/culture/well-being/menopause/people-professionals-guidance
[3]www.menopausecafe.net

Sarah Williams is an Independent Equality, Diversity and Inclusion professional who provides popular EDI and menopause workshops, as well as policy development support. Following her own experiences of chemical and surgical menopause, and seeking support for PMDD, Sarah developed an interest in advocating for menopause inclusion at work and for raising awareness in the community. This has become Sarah's main focus of work. Sarah is also a seasoned facilitator of community peer support and wellbeing groups.

In early 2021, Sarah founded the Menopause Inclusion Collective*, which brings together advocates, activists, menopause professionals and researchers from around the UK to advocate for, and create inclusive menopause policies, projects, resources, services and spaces.

If you would like to connect, we can meet in the Twittersphere: @SarahLouInclude and you can also find me at: www.equalitycounts.co.uk as well as
*www.menopausecollective.org

Printed in Great Britain
by Amazon